Jens Gundgaard

The Distribution of Health and Health Care

An analysis of socio-economic and health-related determinants in a Danish county

University Press of Southern Denmark 2008

© The author and University Press of Southern Denmark 2008

ISBN 987-87-7674-330-7
ISSN 0907-600x

Printed by University of Southern Denmark

Ph.d. dissertation
Faculty of Social Sciences
University of Southern Denmark

Foreword

This thesis presents the result of three years work at the Health Economics Research Unit at the Institute of Public Health, University of Southern Denmark, Odense. The work on the Ph.D. thesis was partly financed by a grant from Faculty of Social Sciences at University of Southern Denmark and partly financed by Centre for Applied Health Services Research and Technology Assessment (CAST), University of Southern Denmark.

The thesis is about the distribution of health and health care. This is in my opinion an interesting topic as it is one aspect of the larger question: What principles should we follow when we allocate scarce resources in the health care sector to comply with efficiency and equity concerns? However, the thesis does not attempt to answer this universal question. It settles for the less ambitious one: How is health and health care actually distributed in Denmark with respect to socio-economic groups?

How health and health care *should* be distributed is a normative question, but how health and health care *are* distributed in an actual society is a positive question that deserves an empirical examination. Although this kind of topic is often laden with implicit normative intentions I have done my best to be objective in all decisions regarding choice of methodology, analysis, and interpretation.

I developed the idea for this research question when it was suggested by fellow researchers from Research Centre for Quality in Medicine Use (FKL) that I should carry out an analysis about the distribution of utilization of medicine across socio-economic groups. During the data collection process I realized that I could get access to data for a range of health care services. I decided to expand the focus of the analysis to include health services at somatic hospitals and in the primary care sector. As the ultimate aim of using health care services is to improve health it was natural also to analyze the distribution of health across socio-economic groups.

The thesis consists of an introduction to the topic, five published articles and one working paper, and a discussion section and a conclusion. Chapter 1 is the introduction to the topic with sections on theories of distributional justice, health behaviour, methodological issues of measurement, and a presentation of the data. In Chapters 2 through 6 the empirical results are presented. Chapter 7 is a paper on the problems of non-response in the data set. An overall discussion of the results, limitations and future research will be found in Chapter 8.

I am indebted to several people for their help during the process of writing the thesis. I would like to thank my supervisor Terkel Christiansen for valuable comments and discussions. I would also like to thank my co-authors on various articles: Jørgen Lauridsen from University of Southern Denmark, Ola Ekholm and Niels Kr. Rasmussen from the National Institute of Public Health, and Ebba Holme Hansen from Copenhagen University.

I am indebted to CAST and head of department Jan Sørensen for helping me with raising funds for half of the Ph.D. project. I am furthermore grateful to Morten Andersen and Jesper Hallas for the provision of prescription records from the OPED database, and to Funen County and Odense University Hospital for delivery of hospital data. I would like to thank Andrew Leach for making it possible for me to go to Canada as a visiting scholar at HEC Montréal and CIRANO, Montreal, Canada, and I would also like to thank Jason Schreiber for proofreading parts of the thesis.

Last but not least, I would like to express my gratitude to my colleagues at the Health Economics Research Unit, CAST, and FKL for being good colleagues and my friends and family for support and encouragement.

Odense, Denmark Jens Gundgaard
March 2008

Table of contents

		page
Chapter 1.	Introduction	6
Chapter 2.	Income related inequality in prescription drugs in Denmark	106
Chapter 3.	Income-related inequality in utilization of health services in Denmark: Evidence from Funen County	134
Chapter 4.	Explaining the sources of income-related inequality in health care utilization in Denmark	157
Chapter 5.	A decomposition of income-related health inequality applied to EQ-5D	180
Chapter 6.	Decomposition of sources of income-related health inequality applied on SF-36 summary scores: a Danish health survey	199
Chapter 7.	The effect of non-response on estimates of health care utilization: The use of health surveys and registers	215
Chapter 8.	Discussion and conclusion	233
	Dansk sammenfatning (Danish summary)	265

Chapter 1

Introduction

Contents of Chapter 1

INTRODUCTION — 9
Introduction to the thesis — 9
Concepts and definitions — 11

THEORIES OF JUSTICE IN HEALTH AND HEALTH CARE — 14
Utilitarianism — 14
Libertarianism — 15
Rawls's theory of justice — 16
Egalitarian theories — 18
Equal treatment for equal need — 18
Equal access for equal need — 19
Equal health — 21
Reward for merit — 22
Concluding remarks — 23

HEALTH BEHAVIOUR — 25
The Grossman model — 25
Comparative statics — 28
Socio-demographic variables — 29
Socio-economic variables — 30
Life-style variables — 32
Some Limitations of the Grossman model — 33
Policy implications of the Grossman Model — 35

MEASURING DISTRIBUTIONAL INEQUALITY OR INEQUITY — 38
Operationalization of definitions — 38

Measuring inequality 39

The concentration index 40
Properties of the concentration index 43
Interpretation of the concentration index in terms of redistribution 46
Inequality aversion in the concentration index 47
Alternative measures 48

Standardizing the concentration index 51

MATERIAL AND SETTING 56

Setting 56
The Danish health care system 56
Objectives of the Danish health care system 58
Funen County 59

The data set 61
Survey data 61
Register based data 64
Health care variables 68
Health variables 69
Standardizing variables 70
Socio-economic variables 71
Life-style variables 74
Study design 74

GUIDE TO THE EMPIRICAL ANALYSES 75

APPENDIX: DESCRIPTIVE STATISTICS 77

REFERENCES 88

Introduction

Introduction to the thesis

Among policy-makers, health professionals, and the general public distributional concerns play an important part of health policy and the organization of the health care sector.[1-5] This thesis is an empirical investigation of the distribution of health and health care in the Danish population. The purpose is to analyze income-related inequality in health and health care in Funen County, Denmark in 2000 and 2001. Concentration indices will be used to characterize the distribution of health and health care with respect to income, and decomposition techniques will be applied to the indices to obtain information about the composition and sources of inequality from determinants and dimensions.

There are potentially many different, and often conflicting, objectives in the health care sector. First of all, health care is meant to improve health and relieve ill-health. By health economists this is most often translated into an efficiency problem with the aim of maximizing health or net benefits in the population.[6] However, the costs and benefits of health and health care can be distributed in numerous ways, and often there is also an objective of distributing health or health care in a way that is perceived just. In almost all health care systems there are elements of public intervention to secure that some sort of equitable concerns are met. But why is it that distributional justice plays such a crucial role in the health care sector? Are the distributional principles to be used in the health care sector different from the distributional principles that are used in the society in general?

Tobin recognized that there are certain specific goods, such as civil rights, basic necessities and health care, that are thought (by the general public as well as policy makers) to be distributed less unequally than the general income distribution in the society. This view was called *specific egalitarianism*.[7] For health care it would mean that treatment of the individual should depend more on medical conditions and less on ability or willingness to pay. Elster has used the concept *local justice* which characterizes good-specific distributive principles that are 1) designed by relatively autonomous institutions, such as health care institutions, 2) only partially compensatory (health care compensates only for health problems), and 3) typically in-kind transfers (health care).[8] Musgrave used the term *merit wants* to characterize public preferences for goods that would be consumed in undesirable quantities, even if there were no market imperfections.[9] Health care could be such a *merit good* where individual consumer sovereignty should be set aside or at least be interfered with to satisfy *merit wants*. According to Daniels, health care is a special good that requires special distributional concerns.[10] He argues that health care is not merely a consumer good like cars or personal computers. Health care is fundamental for restoring and maintaining normal species functioning, such that individuals can maintain a normal range of opportunities of pursuing biological goals as social animals. Culyer et al. have argued that good health is a necessity for the individual to "flourish" as a human being.[11] This provides a justification for treating health care as a special good, although health care is not the only input in the production of good health.

If health care is a special good that requires special distributional arrangements then the policy implications depend on the sources of the motivation for distributional policies. Distributional arrangements can be motivated by altruism or social justice.[1,12] Altruism is rooted in preferences for the well-being of other people. There can be externalities from health, such that the ill-health of sick people contributes negatively in other people's utility functions, due to the possibility that people care about other people's well-being. Furthermore, people might obtain utility by the activity per se of helping others or contributing to the benefit of sick people. As the motivation of altruism is a matter of preferences this approach is ultimately a question of efficiency, and the optimal solution depends on how much preference people have for helping sick people. In principle, the altruistic motive can be built into the economist's efficiency problem of maximizing net benefit of the individuals in the population. The other approach, social justice, is about the commitment to some principles about what is fair and equitable independently of externalities and efficiency. Usually the equitable solution is perceived to be one that is determined by an impartial stance, such that the derived principles are not influenced by individual interests and privileges. The consequences of using the second approach is that efficiency and equity are two separate objectives that may be in conflict with each other, such that the policy makers have to choose between them or to trade-off one with the other.[5,13]

According to Sen, theories of justice usually require that "something" is equal. However, it is less clear what it is that ought to be equal. It is not necessarily health or health care but could also be dimensions such as utilities, rights and liberties.[14,15] The next section will sort out definitions of concepts and principles in theories of justice in the health care sector. This is followed by sections where various theories of justice, applied to health and health care, are presented. A section introduces the economic approach to individual health behaviour and its distributional consequences, and this is followed by a section on empirical measurement methods with a special focus on the concentration index. In the last section of the chapter the data for the empirical investigation are presented, and this section will be completed with a guide to the empirical analyses that are presented in Chapters 2 through 7.

Concepts and definitions

That it is not straightforward to choose Sen's "something" is reflected in the multitude of definitions and interpretations of equity.[11,16-20] First of all, equity is different from equality.[21,22] Whereas equality is a descriptive term characterizing how equal or uniform a distribution of something is, equity is a normative term explaining how fair or just a distribution or a procedure is, relative to some specified norm. Usually, however, as Sen has pointed out, "something" has to be equal to be equitable.

Equity can be interpreted in terms of horizontal and vertical equity.[12,22-25] Horizontal equity is about treating equal individuals (or groups of individuals) equally. To use this concept a definition of relevant characteristics for classifying people as equals is necessary. This means that irrelevant characteristics (with respect to classifying people as equals) should not influence the treatment decision. Vertical equity is about treating unequal individuals (or groups of individuals) unequally. That is, the treatment of unequals should be in appropriate proportion to the inequality of the relevant characteristics.

With regard to health care, the question is whether health care is fundamental for an equitable arrangement or whether health care is merely instrumental as a means to improve health.[20,22] If health care is fundamental, we are concerned about either the distribution of health care or the procedures for allocating health care to patients. If health care is instrumental we are only interested in health care insofar as it results in the desirable consequences, namely producing the appropriate amount of health. In fact, health care is usually only consumed for the effect it has on health (or on utility through health). Health care per se is most often perceived as a bad rather than a good.[26] Williams, along the lines of Donabedian, has classified these elements of focus into resources, processes, and outcome.[23,27] The outcome in terms of health (or utility) is a function of the processes of allocating and providing health care which again is a function of the resources put into the system. These chains of elements are constrained downwards such that if the focus is on health outcome certain procedures and allocation mechanisms, as well as available resources, are necessary to achieve the desired equitable distribution of health. If the focus is on the processes, that is, certain procedures for allocating health care, then the resources are constrained to implement these allocation mechanisms. However, the resulting health outcome is not constrained but ends up with whatever the resulting distribution might be. Likewise, if the resources are the focus the unconstrained processes and health outcomes are results of the equitable distribution of resources.

The chain of elements shows the constraints imposed on one level as a consequence of having the focus on another. However, the objective function of what to focus on can be specified and optimized in numerous ways. In mainstream economics the focus is "welfarist".[28] That is, the concern is with utility of the individuals where health is only one factor to influence utility. This puts health care on the same footing as other goods in the objective of increasing utility. Another school of economics is "extra-welfarist".[28] In this branch of health economics it is recognized that the objectives in the health care sector by and large are to improve health (the trade-off between resources to the health care sector and other sectors is carried out elsewhere). Health care is assessed by its instrumentality in producing health. Health is most often seen as a combination of quality of life and length of life (e.g. QALYs).

Other objectives are, of course, possible too. Health care can also be assessed by its instrumentality to bring about opportunities to live a normal life devoid of the constraints from ill-health.[10] Thus, the objective is to optimize opportunities in the society. Opportunities can also be specified with respect to achieving a certain health status.[21]

If the concern is more directed towards the processes the objective function could be constructed to optimize an equitable distribution or allocation mechanism of health care. Furthermore, the focus could also be on less tangible or quantifiable factors such as access to health care [19,20,22] or patient autonomy, for example patient rights and freedom to choose.[29-31]

The objective function can be optimized in several ways[1].[32] If the focus is on a single factor, say health, the objective function can be maximized or equalized, or some mixture of that. If the objective function contains more than one factor, say health and patient rights, there are various solutions that may have quite different policy implications.[32] 1) The two factors can be optimized together by some weights for the importance attached to each of them. 2) If one factor has absolute priority, say patient rights, it can be incorporated as a side-constraint, such that (say) health has to be optimized subject to the constraint of not violating patient rights. 3) The two factors can be optimized lexicographically one by one with two different objective functions with independent optimization procedures.

All these endless possibilities for distributing health and health care open up the question of how to choose the principles for equitable arrangements in the health care sector. One can find inspiration in various theories of justice to answer questions like that. With inspiration from Gillon the theories, have been classified into five categories: Utilitarian theories, libertarian theories, Rawls's theory of justice, egalitarian theories, and reward for merit.[30] These theories will be presented in the next section.

---

[1] The word "optimize" is used in lieu of the word "maximize" to accentuate the fact that simple sum-ranking is not necessarily the desired way of choosing the relevant state.

Theories of justice in health and health care

Utilitarianism

Utilitarian theories developed out of nineteenth-century liberalism represented by Bentham and Mill.[33,34] Three essential elements characterize utilitarianism: 1) It is welfarist, that is, the evaluation is in terms of individual utility. 2) It is consequentialist. This means that utilitarian theory is outcome oriented. The procedures are not important, as long as the consequence is an increase in individual utility. 3) It applies sum ranking: The objective function of utility is optimized by maximizing the sum of individual utility where everyone, according to the Benthamite dictum, counts for one and nobody more than one.[32-35]

In classical utilitarianism utility was synonymous with happiness and interpreted in terms of pleasure and pain. All actions and interventions should be evaluated alone by their tendency to promote pleasure and to avoid pain.[33,34] Mill moderated the concept of utility by interpreting it in the largest sense of the word, and by quality adjusting utility into higher and lower value pleasures, where higher value pleasures are pleasures of the intellect, feelings, and imaginations.[34] While these interpretations of utility can be quite intangible (and normative from the point of view of the policy-maker) utility is by modern utilitarianism interpreted as individuals' preferences; either as the individuals' true, rational preferences if all relevant information was available, or as in economics, where complete consumer sovereignty is assumed, individual's observed preferences.[36,37]

The consequentialist approach implies that only consequences for individual utility ultimately matter. Interpreted strictly, how we achieve the outcome is immaterial. Side-constraints such as personal rights and liberty can in principle be built in, but the justification ultimately rests on the effect on consequences for individual utility.

Sen's "something" that ought to be equal is for utilitarianism the equal weight to everyone in the summation of utility regardless of social position. According to Hare, it is hard to use any other weights than equal weights when impartially allocating benefits and burdens between different people.[38] Following Harsanyi, rational people, not knowing their position in society, would in theory have an equal probability of being in every possible social position. They would in this impartial stance choose to maximize expected utility by letting everyone count as one.[37,39,40] The distribution of utility across individuals per se is irrelevant in utilitarianism. However, due to diminishing marginal utility of most goods, the practical implications will in many cases mean substantial redistribution of goods towards a more uniform distribution of these goods,[38] not because an equal distribution is valued higher but because a more equal distribution is an instrument for maximizing welfare.

Health is one element among others that can increase utility, possibly with diminishing marginal effect, such that health ought to be "redistributed" from people with high health status to people with low health status to maximize overall welfare. However, if some people have little or no chance of improving health, the implication could also be a redistribution of resources to the benefit of the already better-off.

The utilitarian solution is often perceived as being equivalent to the notion of economic efficiency. However, in economic literature it is not always clear whether efficiency corresponds to maximizing utility or Pareto optimality. The utilitarian principles of sum-ranking and consequentialism can also be applied directly on health. These are the principles applied in the extra-welfarist approach to health economic evaluation.

Libertarianism

The libertarian theory is first and foremost concerned with individual rights to liberty and possessions. These rights reflect the Kantian principle that individuals are ends in themselves and not merely means. As individuals' rights are inviolable the rights should therefore be seen as side-constraints in the pursuit of any societal objectives. That is, the rights should not be maximized in utilitarian fashion (not utilitarianism of rights: some rights should not be violated for the sake of complying more with others). Instead they are inviolable for every individual.[41] The violation of rights is also the main concern with the expansion of the state. According to Nozick, only a minimal state that takes care of no more than basic tasks such as securing law and order, enforcement of contracts and private property rights, is compatible with not violating people's rights.[41]

Libertarianism is anti-consequentialist or process-oriented. As long as the holdings of goods are acquired by principles of just acquisition, that is, no rights are violated and transfers have occurred through productive exchange, then the resulting distribution of holdings are just, and people are entitled to these holdings.

Health care is perceived as a good like any other that people can be entitled to according to the principles of just acquisition. Simply because health care is often thought to have an internal goal of improving health it doesn't mean that health care should be allocated on the basis of need for health care. Other goods also have internal goals and they are not (and should not be, according to libertarian theories) allocated according to the need for them.[41] Redistributive schemes, i.e. to reallocate health care, financed by, say, income taxes, would violate individuals' rights as some individuals are used as involuntary means to benefit others. Voluntary donations such as charity to redistribute resources to health care would, on the other hand, be acceptable, as holdings acquired from someone else who is entitled to the holding, would be in agreement with the principle of just acquisition.

In reality, there are advocates of these ideas who support libertarian principles for consequentialist reasons such as the belief that market-oriented solutions are more efficient, or mistrust in government intervention.[42] In less strict versions of libertarianism, it could be a public task to provide some sort of decent minimum of health care.

Rawls's theory of justice

In economics Rawls is known for the maximin-principle which is about distributing goods such that the distribution is to the benefit of the least well-off. Rawls's theory of justice is, of course, more complex than just the maximin-principle. As is true with Harsanyi's thinking, the Rawlsian solution is based on the impartial choice of rational individuals.[43] Rawls asks how rational individuals would choose the principles for distributing advantages, rights and duties in the society if they were placed behind a "veil of ignorance" not knowing their place in society with respect to class, social status, ability and intelligence, but would be aware of the constraints of human psychology and economic principles. According to Rawls, these people would unanimously choose two principles that are to be fulfilled in lexicographical order. 1) Basic liberties such as freedom of speech and assembly, right to vote, and property rights are to be distributed equally and at the highest level. The first principle has to be met before the second. Basic liberties in one area can be traded off only with other basic liberties. 2) The second principle consists of two principles. Public offices and positions have to be open to all given a fair equality of opportunity. Furthermore, (an index of) social primary goods, that is all goods that every rational man is presumed to want - liberties and opportunities, income and wealth, and self-respect - are to be allocated to the benefit of the worst off. That is, an unequal distribution of the index of social primary goods can be justified only if it is to the advantage of the least well-off.[2] This latter principle is what is often called the maximin principle or the difference principle.[43] Other primary goods such as intelligence and imagination, capacities and skills, health and vigor are natural goods, and although they are influenced by allocation principles in the society, they are not directly under its control to be modified.[43]

The least well-off is not supposed to literally mean the worst-off person in the society but rather the group of people in the lowest class or specified to people with some minimum level of primary goods over a life-time.[43,44] In addition, the two principles are not meant to aid micro-level decisions but refer to the structure of the basic institutions in society.

What role does health and health care play in the Rawlsian framework? According to Sen, an equal level of primary goods cannot be enjoyed equally by people with different levels of health status. To simplify things, Rawls has assumed that the rational individuals are fully cooperating members of society in which no one is sick and in need of health care.[45] Applying the difference principle to health would, according to Arrow, potentially degrade the population to poverty, as there can easily exist expensive health care procedures for the worst-off people with little effect.[46] Daniels has argued that health

---

[2] Equivalent to right-angled social indifference curves.

care should not be treated as a social primary good.[10] Instead, it ought to be treated as an integrated part of the basic institutions that promote fair opportunities. Health care institutions are to help bring sick people back to normal functioning so they can pursue biological goals as social animals with the same opportunities as anyone else. This does not mean that health care institutions should be aimed at making health distributed completely equal among people. It means that health care institutions should work on restoring what is normal functioning for these people[3]. Rawls has endorsed this aim of restoring people so they again are fully cooperative members of society.[45]

Egalitarian theories
Egalitarianism is here seen as an umbrella of different theories with the focus on equality in health or health care. This approach has its origin in Marxism, but as pointed out by Wagstaff et al. it has also played an important part of twentieth-century egalitarianism.[12] A number of principles have been suggested for the distribution of health and health care.

Equal treatment for equal need
Absolute equality in health care has rarely been suggested as the egalitarian principle at an individual level. However, across geographical regions within a country, there is often some equalization in expenditures or resources available. At an individual level it would in most cases not be considered appropriate if a sizable fraction of the health care budget was allocated to people who were in no need of health care. That is, it would be considered more fair if need was taken into account in the allocation procedure[4]. The challenge with this definition is that it rests on the definition of need. Need is seen as something different from demand.[22] Whereas demand is what is desired by the individual, given prices, need is seen as something

---

[3] Health care is compared with education where it is suggested that there should be equal opportunities for equal skills and aspirations. For practical implementation equal access for equal need is advocated.
[4] As in the second half of the Marxian dictum of "From each according to his ability – to each according to his needs".

objectively measurable by a third-party independently of what is desired by the individual. There can possibly be demand without need and vice versa. However, need for health care still has several possible definitions, each with distinctive policy implications. In general, they will not lead to equality in health, unless people are identical. Usually need is perceived as *severity of illness*. The more severe a person's ill-health is the more he needs health care. Using severity as a principle for the allocation of health care has been criticized as a severely ill person hardly can be said to need health care if he cannot benefit from it. Instead, need can be interpreted as *capacity to benefit* from health care. This means that health care should be allocated in proportion to the capacity to benefit. However, capacity to benefit might appear discriminatory to very sick people with little capacity to benefit. Indeed, if met marginally the principle is identical to the utilitarian solution applied to health. Nevertheless, if the benefits are interpreted as utilities the principle is moderated somewhat as even a small increment in health status for the sick may result in a huge increase in utility[5]. Alternatively, the resources can be taken into account by defining need as *the resources required to exhaust capacity to benefit*. This way more health care is needed for a person who requires more health care to achieve his maximum possible health status whether the capacity to benefit is large or small.

Equal access for equal need
Many researchers and policy makers find the principle of equal treatment for equal need too paternalistic. Patients in equal need, regardless of the definition, might not have the same preferences for utilizing health care as the effect on health is far from the only input in people's utility functions. To also respect people's autonomy, the advocated principle by many policy documents and researchers is *equal access for equal need*.[19,20] Access is, of course, an intangible concept that also requires some definition. Often the concept has caused some confusion as some researchers have taken it to mean realized access, that is, actual utilization, and by others it is taken to mean options or opportunities to use.[20,47] To use the latter definition equal access can

---

[5] Assuming diminishing marginal utility of health.

be defined in terms of equal prices for health care faced by the patients. However, most often *and free access* is added to *equal access* to ensure that by access is meant prices at zero or almost zero for health care services at the point of delivery of health care, such that the patients are free to use health care services in proportion to the specified definition of need. However, many barriers can still exist for health care prices at zero. There can be transport costs and opportunity costs of spending time away from work to utilize health care services that would have to be equalized or compensated for to ensure equal opportunities[6].[48] Olsen et al. have defined equal access as a situation where people are able to consume the same quantity of health care services.[49] If the maximum possible level of consumption should be equal across individuals with different incomes it means that the prices (and possibly also other costs) of health care should vary with incomes. However, the level of health care utilization will not necessarily be the same for people with different incomes even for people with the same preferences as the trade-offs with other goods would be different.[11] Health care prices at zero would make the consumption of other goods independent of consumption of health care. If income is influenced by time (to work), the opportunity costs would still be different for individuals with the same preferences. One solution would be to make the choice sets identical for all individuals. That would, however, remove the status of health care as a special good that needs special attention and change it to a good among all other goods that could be purchased for equalized incomes across individuals. The analyses could be further complicated by treating the cost in utility terms. Assuming decreasing marginal utility of income, the richer people would have to pay more for equal loss in utility for consuming health care. Introducing utility as the unit of measurement would require interpersonal utility comparisons. In addition, using utility also opens up the possibility of including process utility as a cost or benefit of the access per se, or process utility as a cost or benefit of consuming the health care services.[50]

---

[6] Perhaps the relevant price is the shadow price of health. This definition of price will be applied in the section on health behaviour.

Equal health

A number of researchers think that utilization or access is only valuable for the instrumentality of producing health. That is, the first and foremost aim of the health care sector should be equality in health. Although this objective seems simpler at first sight, a number of questions also arise here. Equalizing health completely would probably only be possible by lowering the average level of health considerably as some people are incurably sick. Still, as a trade-off with efficiency objectives, the principle could be implemented by giving lower weight to health gains of people with higher health status compared with lower health status. Consequently, the variation in health status will not be minimized but only restrained.

Another, and to a certain degree, related question is to what extent health inequalities between people from different socio-demographic groups, such as age and gender, are acceptable[7].[51,52] According to Daniels, it should not be considered discriminatory to favour some age groups more than others as everybody ages. The age criterion operates in principle within lives and not between lives and should be perceived as prudent redistribution across a lifetime. Favouring some age groups over others would therefore not violate the Kantian dictum of treating people as means per se, and not merely as ends.

Williams has advocated the *fair innings* argument which is based on the view that it is more tragic when a young person dies than when and old person dies.[2,23,53] The basic assumption is that everybody is entitled to some "normal" length of (quality adjusted) life – a fair innings. This implies that young people, who have not already had their fair innings should, *ceteris paribus*, have priority over older people who have had a long (quality adjusted) life. A variant of the fair innings argument has been suggested by Stolk et al., who have suggested the *proportional shortfall*. This principle is about giving priority to people on the basis of their expected loss of future quality adjusted time relative to their remaining life expectancy.[54,55] The principle is an attempt to combine the *fair innings* argument and the *severity of illness*. The introduction of the *fair innings* argument and the

---

[7] Obviously, there are "natural" differences in health between socio-demographic groups, but that is also the case within socio-demographic groups.

proportional shortfall necessitates the distinction between retrospective and prospective health.[56] Normally economics is forward looking and perceive retrospective costs and benefits as "sunk". With the *fair innings* argument a natural question arise about whether health equality should be about future health alone, e.g. equality in future health or future health gains, or whether health equality should aim at equality in overall health gains including past gains.

Reward for merit

In the utilitarian approach everybody counts for one, and nobody more than one. A variant of this approach is that some count more than others because they are more deserving. This desert could originate from, among other things, contribution to society such as military service, participation in the labour market, tax contributions, being the breadwinner of a family, or with reverse sign, criminal behaviour.[30,32] The merit related criteria can be backward looking, i.e. reward for past behaviour, or forward looking, i.e. to achieve future contributions.[30]

Although there are not many proponents of the reward for merit principle among researchers, some elements of forward looking merits can be found in economic evaluation and actual micro-rationing in the health care sector.[24] With respect to backward looking merits they are mainly to be found when it comes to health choices. Ill-health is, for example by Le Grand, regarded as inequitable if it is outside of the control of the individual.[21] If the ill-health results from factors with the individual's control, then it is considered acceptable. Factors within the individual's control could be life-style choices such as smoking or heavy drinking. Health inequalities due to voluntary chosen unhealthy life-styles are therefore not considered inequitable. To secure that everybody has access to health care, the individuals with unhealthy choices should be compelled to pay a risk premium (in addition to general tax or social insurance contributions) in proportion to the additional risk of their voluntary risky choices.

The principles suggested by Le Grand belong to a class of theories that stresses equality in opportunities. Sen has introduced the concepts of *functionings* and *capability*[8].[14,15,57] Where *capability* is what a person can actually do (like a budget constraint of *functionings*) the *functionings* are the actual achievements consisting of beings and doings such as being in good health, being happy, having self-respect. People with the same set of *capabilities* may choose different bundles of *functionings*. To Sen, health equity is a multidimensional concept including concerns about achievements of health as well as capabilities to achieve health. Furthermore, Sen has recognized that processes are also important for equitably distributing health care.

Concluding remarks

The previous section has given a brief review of the most influential theories of justice applied to health and health care. It is obvious that there are many competing claims for the definition of just health care, and evidently some of these claims can be in conflict with each other. Nevertheless, there will also be many situations where some of the claims will coincide, such as situations where, for instance, the most severely ill person is also the one with the biggest capacity to benefit, and the most efficient one to treat from the point of view of maximizing overall health and minimizing health inequality. However, it is easy to imagine situations where this will not be the case.

The question is whether there should be a single equity principle to guide all decisions in the health care sector, or whether different norms and standards should be applied at different levels or in different contexts. Actual decision-making is probably closer to the latter than the former. Health care resources are allocated though numerous decisions at various levels ranging from the national level regarding the overall budget to the clinical decision-making level concerning the individual patient. There are various reasons why we do not have a *de facto* single over-arching principle applied to all levels and contexts. (1) People are context specific and have different equity perceptions in different situations.[6,32] (2) Even if people were not context specific per se, they might not agree with each other, and in the decision-making process it might be impossible to decide on a single

---

[8] It is inequitable to classify Sen in the *Reward for merit* category. However, his health equity concept fits into the discussion of choice.

principle. (3) Having different norms and standards at different levels is one way of trading-off different concerns; e.g. if we prefer not to discriminate between individuals at the clinical level we can choose to implement health care interventions at a national or regional level that will, on average, benefit some groups of individuals more than others without discriminating at the individual level.[58] (4) Having a complicated decision-making process at different levels probably also serves the purpose to mask the simple truth that uncomfortable decisions have to be made when resources are scarce.[59]

What is the economist's role in all this? What equity principles to follow is, of course, a normative question, and the economist should in general be no better (or worse) than anyone else in suggesting what is equitable and what is not. The economist might, however, to a larger degree be able to point out the consequences of choosing certain principles and evaluate the effects of trading off principles with each other.[6,23,32] Although a transparent quantification of the consequences of different principles would be in conflict with (4) it would make it easier to assess if a policy is in accordance with chosen or suggested equity principles.

Health Behaviour

The Grossman model

The previous sections introduced the normative principles of how to distribute health and health care. The actual implementation of allocation principles is, of course, restricted by health behaviour and the health production relations. In this section an economic approach is chosen to explain some aspects of health behaviour that can lead to differences in health and health care across population groups. Economics treats groups as sets of individuals with the same characteristics. The strategy is therefore to analyze the effect of these characteristics on individual behaviour. The economic approach is inspired by Grossman's pioneering work from 1972 on demand for health.[60,61]

In Grossman's model, health has nearly the same properties as a durable capital good. Investments in health improve the health status, in economic terms the health stock, but over time the health stock also depreciates. Another interesting feature is that the investments in health take place as a production with health care and time as inputs. The consumer doesn't simply demand health care. Demand for health care is derived demand for health investments. Likewise, the demand for other market goods is also a derived demand for the production of what is here called *commodities*, that is, leisure activities that can be produced with market goods and time as inputs. The demand for health is, as all other goods, determined by price. The relevant price for health is the shadow price, which depends on several variables and not merely on the costs of health care alone, and it is negatively related with health demanded.[60,61]

If uncertainty is not introduced into the model the consumer chooses his length of life by deciding how much to invest in health given the restrictions from the production relations. Health is demanded for two reasons: 1) partly for the investment aspect. Good health produces more time without illness, that is, more healthy days, which can be used to produce more commodities (or more accurately, a higher budget set that can be spent on leisure and market goods in the production of commodities), 2) and partly for the consumption aspect, that is, utility is obtained directly from time being in good health.[60,61]

The individual's utility can therefore be expressed as a function of commodities and healthy time:

$$U = U(Z_0,...,Z_n, f(H_0),..., f(H_n)), \qquad (1)$$

where Z_i is spending on commodities and $f(H_i)$ is the production of healthy time in the ith period, respectively. Healthy time h_i in period i is produced by the health stock H_i through $f(H_i)$ which is a concave function as healthy time is naturally limited by the number of days in a given year.

A person's health stock in a given period is determined by the health stock in the previous period plus the gross investment in health in the previous period I_{i-1} and minus the depreciation of the health stock by the depreciation rate δ_{i-1} as health naturally deteriorates if nothing is done to maintain it.

$$H_i = H_{i-1} + I_{i-1} - \delta_{i-1} H_{i-1}. \qquad (2)$$

Investments in health and commodities are produced by

$$I_i = I_i(M_i, T_{Hi}; E_i)$$
$$Z_i = Z_i(X_i, T_{Zi}; E_i), \qquad (3)$$

where M_i is health care, T_{Hi} is time spent on health improving activities such as exercise or time to receive health care services. X_i is market goods purchased and T_{Zi} is time spent on leisure activities.[9] E_i is the human capital component for how efficient I_i and Z_i are produced. In this model E_i is unrelated to the health status and exogenously determined (However, in reality the health stock and human capital stock would probably be correlated for some values of the stocks).

The consumer's optimization problem is to maximize the utility function subject to a budget constraint. The budget constraint is how the present value of consumption of health care, market goods and time spent on health improving activities, on producing commodities, and on ill-health (healthy days lost) are constrained by the present value of the full wealth, that is the value of the maximum hours worked plus initial wealth:

---

[9] Constant returns to scale production functions have been chosen for simplicity.

$$\sum \frac{P_{Mi}M_i + P_{Xi}X_i + W_i(T_{Hi} + T_{Zi} + T_{Li})}{(1+r)^i} = \sum \frac{W_i \Omega}{(1+r)^i} + A_0, \qquad (4)$$

where P_{Mi} and P_{Xi} are the prices of health care and market goods, W_i the wage rate, Ω the number of hours in a year, and A_0 initial wealth (such as inheritance).

Formula 1 and 4 can be used in a Langrangian function. By focusing only on the health choice in one period the first order condition can be found with respect to the health investment variable I_{i-1}. Taking into account the first order condition with respect to health investments in period i and rearranging we obtain the central optimality condition in Grossman's model:

$$MP_{Hi}\left[\frac{W_i}{MC_{Ii-1}} + \frac{MU_{hi}}{\lambda MC_{Ii-1}}(1+r)^i\right] = r + \partial_i - M\dot{C}_{Ii-1}, \qquad (5)$$

which says that the marginal benefit of health capital must equal the marginal costs of health capital. The left-hand-side of the optimality condition expresses the value of the marginal product of health capital MP_{Hi}. The first term in the brackets is the pecuniary valuation of the health capital weighted by the marginal costs of investments MC_{Ii-1}[10]. The second term in the brackets refers to the direct returns from health. MU_{hi} is the direct marginal utility from healthy days weighted by the Lagrangian multiplier λ (which is to be interpreted as the marginal utility of wealth) and the marginal costs of investments. The right-hand-side of the optimality condition represents the user costs of health capital. r is the interest rate and corresponds to the opportunity costs of holding capital, δ_i is the depreciation rate and denotes the costs of deterioration, and the last term on the right-hand-side, $M\dot{C}_{Ii-1}$, represents what Grossman calls capital gains, which is a component of changes in the cost of investment in percentage terms.[60] Health capital is non-tradable in that it cannot be sold or rented out in a market. However, as Grossman explains, by lowering or increasing investments over periods, one can rent capital from oneself by redistributing health capital over periods.

---

[10] To follow Grossman's exposition and express the shadow price in relative terms the marginal costs of investments have been moved from the right-hand-side to the left-hand-side. Still, it should be kept in mind that the marginal cost is really a supply-side phenomenon.

Comparative statics

Given the possibility that there are two aspects of investing in health — the investment aspect and the consumption aspect — separate comparative statics analyses are often carried out for the two aspects with most of the weight given to the investment aspect. A justification for separate analyses can be the assumption that direct effects on health are small compared to the pecuniary effects such that the pecuniary effects are interesting per se[11].[62] The pecuniary effect should not be interpreted literally as utility obtained from income. Rather, it represents utility obtained from *commodities*, which are seen as a wider representation of activities produced with leisure time and market goods. If the direct marginal utility from health time MU_{hi} is zero then formula 5 reduces to:

$$\frac{MP_{Hi}W_i}{MC_{Ii-1}} = r + \partial_i - \dot{MC}_{Ii-1}. \tag{6}$$

The left-hand side is then the pecuniary benefits of the health stock. Since the number of produced healthy days is limited by the number of days in the year the marginal efficiency of additional investments in health is decreasing (but with a decreasing rate). This demand curve for health capital is shown in Figure 1. The right-hand side, the user cost of capital, is represented by the supply curve in Figure 1. As the user cost of capital is uncorrelated with the stock of capital the supply curve is perfectly elastic.[60] Likewise, if the focus is on the consumption aspect, the optimality condition can be approximated by equating the consumption part of the right-hand side of formula 5 with the user cost of capital:

$$\frac{MP_{Hi}MU_{hi}}{\lambda MC_{Ii-1}}(1+r)^i = r + \partial_i - \dot{MC}_{Ii-1}. \tag{7}$$

As can be seen from formula 7 a wealth effect — Lagrangian multiplier λ — enters into the optimality condition which was not the case in the investment part of the model. For the consumption aspect the demand behaviour over time is not determined by the efficiency of capital but by

---

[11] Obviously, the technical convenience of separate analyses also plays a role for this choice.

the intertemporal preferences between present and future health.[61] The following sections will illuminate the possible effect of different types of variables on health behaviour.

Figure 1. Supply and demand for health capital

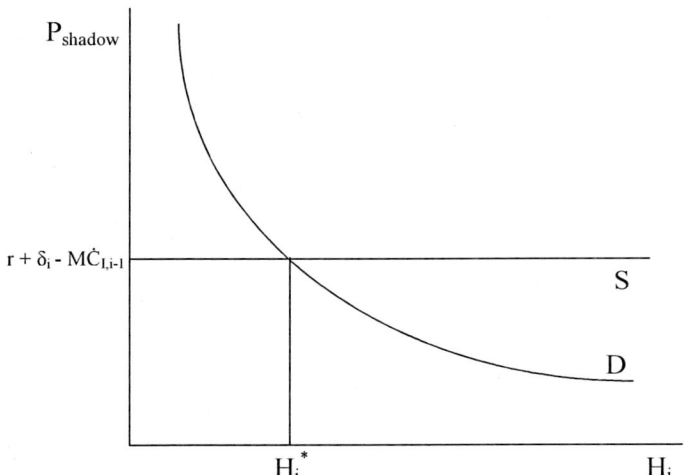

Socio-demographic variables

Presumably the depreciation rate increases with age. At least after a certain age the consumer's health will deteriorate. The consumer will die when his health stock is below a certain level H_{min}. The consumer can offset the deterioration by investing more in health. In the investment model the more inelastic demand is the more investments will take place to offset a unit's decrease in the health stock. As a person ages the supply curve moves upwards when the depreciation rate increases. When the demand is inelastic the gross investments in health will increase, such that decreasing health status will be observed at the same time as increasing health investments, e.g. higher utilization of health care. As the depreciation rate becomes too high the consumer will not be able to off-set the deterioration in health as it simply becomes too costly to do so. When the health stock has fallen to below H_{min} the consumer dies. The consumer chooses the length of life which is in accordance with maximizing the present value of consumption of *commodities* and that is not necessarily the maximum length of life[12].[60,61]

In the consumption model the consumer will also choose a finite length of life as investing in the health stock in the end becomes too costly with a rising depreciation rate. However, the intertemporal preferences allows the consumer to increase net investments over some parts of the life cycle with increasing depreciation rates at the expense of lower health stocks in other periods.[61,62]

Gender is not treated explicitly in the Grossman model. There are, of course, biological differences between men and women. Possibly the depreciation rates could be thought to change with different patterns over the life course, although it is not easy to model how. Furthermore, there could be some indirect effects through the socio-economic variables (position in the labour market, educational status etc., and these effects are handled in the next section). It is also quite possible that women have different preferences than men, but this will be reflected in the consumption model only.

Socio-economic variables

The relevant socio-economic variables for the present analyses are income, education, occupation, and marital status. Formal income is represented by the wage rate W_i in the Grossman model as income is generated by time spent on work for wages (informal income can be generated by the household production function). In the investment model, a higher wage rate will imply a higher value of the marginal product of health capital. The marginal costs of investing in health will also increase as time will become more expensive. However, as health is produced by both time and health care, this effect is smaller than the wage effect and an increase in the wage rate will be equivalent to an outward shift in the demand curve in Figure 1. This results in a higher equilibrium health capital stock. In other words, individuals from the

---

[12] A higher present value is always preferable to a lower present value regardless of personal intertemporal preferences (with perfect capital markets. However, in real life capital markets are far from perfect and life cycle redistribution might be easier for some groups than others).

higher income groups have an incentive to invest more in health and to be healthier as they have higher opportunity costs of being away from work due to illness. In the consumption part of the model, the result is more unclear as higher wages make it more expensive to invest in health as well as to produce commodities.[60,61]

Education enters into the model as the human capital component, E_i, in the production functions from formula (3). It is hypothesized that higher educated people are more efficient producers of health (That is, lower marginal costs MC_{Ii-1} for the same level of production). Perhaps they are more aware of the importance of life-style choices or simply better producers of the inputs in the production of health[13]. In the investment part of the model a higher level of education will simply make the health capital more efficient equivalent to shifting the demand curve to the right. A higher level of education would make health more profitable and increase demand for health capital. However, if the demand curve is elastic, which it is for healthy consumers, then more education could increase the demand for health but at the same time decrease the demand for health care.[60,61] If human capital had an effect on the wage rate, which is the normal assumption in human capital models but is ignored for simplicity in the Grossman model, there would also be an indirect effect through higher income.

In the consumption model, things are more complicated as the introduction of the wealth effect in the optimality condition creates two possible off-setting effects: a wealth effect and a substitution effect.

Occupational status is a more intangible variable to handle at an abstract level as it is more multifaceted and can barely be analyzed as one variable. A few aspects will be mentioned here. If manual work requires more wear and tear on the body, then that could be equivalent to a higher depreciation rate.[63] From an investment perspective that would make it less profitable to invest in health capital: The user cost of capital would become more expensive and the supply curve would move upwards. People with physically hard work would tend to choose a shorter life, as it would simply be too expensive to live long, given the other good things in life[14]. Another aspect of occupational status is the

---

[13] Such as knowing how to take medicine or following advice from the physician.
[14] Stressful or mentally hard work could have the same effect on the depreciation rate.

labour force participation. People outside the labour market would normally have a lower income, typically given as transfers or informal income produced by the household production function[15]. Given the assumption of lower income the effect is as described earlier for individuals with lower wages compared to individuals with higher wages. That is, people outside the labour market are expected to aim for a lower stock of health. In general, there are some indirect effects of occupational status. For many jobs there is an element of human capital production that would affect the size of E_i, and obviously the wage rate W_i is also attached to the type of job.

The last socio-economic variable mentioned is the marital status variable. Although somewhat speculative, one can hypothesize that being divorced or widowed is stressful and is hard on the health and that these states have higher depreciation rates than being married or single. Statuses such as being married or single are probably too diverse for any predictions in the Grossman model.

Life-style variables

Health behaviour is often connected with life-style factors such as smoking, alcohol consumption, diet and exercises. The simplest way to treat the life-style variables in the theoretical framework is to assume that unhealthy life-style is simply lack of investment in health, and by the same token, a healthy life-style is equivalent to higher gross investments. That is, life-style choices are endogenously determined. The lower income groups have a lower incentive to invest in good health for the various reasons explained above, and that might also be reflected in life-style choices such as smoking, alcohol consumption, diet and exercises. That is, even with perfect information about the health consequences, it might be perfectly rational for the lower socio-economic groups to pay less attention to living a healthy life.[63]

Another way the life-style choices might be affected is through the human capital component, which is exogenously determined. With less than perfect information it might be plausible that

---

[15] It is, of course, plausible that people have chosen to stay outside the labour market because they are more efficient producers of informal income than what can be earned in the labour market.

the higher educated have more knowledge on the health effects of lifestyle choices or how to implement them in real life. In that sense lifestyle choices could simply be a part of the human capital component as a practical implementation of a more efficient production technology.

Some Limitations of the Grossman model

The Grossman model assumes that decisions are made with perfect certainty of outcomes.[62] This means that the consumer can choose his own health state given the biological and economic restriction and in principle determine his length of life. Given the fact that health is highly stochastic it might be an unreasonable assumption. The most obvious way to incorporate uncertainty in the model is to assume a known or unknown probability distribution for the depreciation rate. Most likely such a distribution would be left-skewed in the sense that the depreciation rate would cluster closely around a mean depreciation rate most of the time with some rare upward fluctuations big enough for even the healthiest consumer to die unexpectedly from one period to the next. According to Grossman, the risk-averse consumer will invest more in good health in order to offset the possible loss in income due to randomly low depreciation rates the following years.[62] There are, however, probably also effects in the other direction as future consumption will be lost due to sudden death, which will increase the incentive for the risk-averse consumer to invest less in health and spend more on commodities sooner than later. How this would affect health investments across socio-economic groups depends on the probability distribution and the risk-aversion of the different groups and the magnitudes of the different off-setting effects[16].

Another assumption in the Grossman model is that the consumer has perfect information about the production relations. Although the consumer might be well-informed about household production it would most often be necessary to rely on expert opinions about the effects of health investments and, perhaps also, the depreciation rate. The consequence of relying on expert judgment depends on the agency relationship, that is, to what degree the physician

---

[16] Many of the extensions to the Grossman model are about how uncertainty can be incorporated formally into the model.[64-67]

works as a perfect agent for the patient (the consumer).[68] According to Culyer, the perfect agent is the one who would suggest actions that the patient would have chosen himself had he had the same informational advantages as the physician.[28] In that case the agency relationship would not put any constraints on individual behaviour suggested by the Grossman model. However, in some situations the agency relationship might not be perfect. Even if the physician does his best to be a perfect agent it might be impossible for the physician to transfer information perfectly to the patient or to obtain information about patient preferences from the patient such that the physician can make decisions on behalf of the patient.[69,70] Furthermore, the physician does not always have an incentive to be a perfect agent. Although constrained by medical codes of ethics, physicians have in many situations an incentive to induce demand to a higher level than the patient would have chosen had he had the same information as the physician (supplier-induced demand).[71,72] If the remuneration systems are set such that more services are correlated with a higher income for the physician there is definitely a motive and an incentive for the physician to induce more demand for health care than the patient would have chosen with full information.[73] So if supplier-induced demand does take place, at least to some extent, the consumer will invest more in health than would otherwise be the case (or they will demand health services that may or may not have an improvement of health).[74] With respect to this thesis, the question is how an imperfect agency relationship will influence behaviour across socio-economic groups. One could hypothesize that the agency relationship would be less perfect for people with a lower human capital component. Perhaps it would be easier to induce demand for people who would have less information about the health production relations.[68,75] If these people are more in contact with the health care sector (perhaps they invest more in health care to partly offset a higher depreciation rate) it might be easier for physicians to find services where demand can be induced. At least it is more difficult to induce demand for people who are rarely in contact with the health care system. However, in a system with free services at the point of delivery people with more information, such as consumers with a higher human capital component, might on the other hand be more successful in inducing supply (demand-induced supply)[17]. That is, the well-informed consumers may be more persistent and more skilled in negotiating more services from the physician[18].[68,75] It seems that there are several off-setting effects of the agency relationship and the actual effect on health behaviour is an empirical question[19]. The theory of the agency relationship, however, does tell us that demand for health investment such as health care utilization might not be completely separated from supply of these services, and this relationship most likely influences the demand for some groups more than others.[76]

Another limitation is the fact that the Grossman model only attempts to explain the aspects of health behaviour that is determined by the rational considerations about optimizing well-being over a life cycle. Although a high degree of human behaviour is controlled by rational thoughtfulness, human behaviour is also, to a high degree, determined by cultural norms and habits, group behaviour and peer pressure shaped by the social environment, as well as coincidences, and limited information and understandings of health.[77-81] People do not in all situations think about how different types of health behaviour will work as investments in health to maximize utility over a life course. However, as an approximation of the choice of life-style in general, the model might have enough predictive power to explain at least some important aspects of health behaviour.

Policy implications of the Grossman Model

What we can learn from the Grossman model, despite some of its limitations, is that it would often be rational or optimal for people in different circumstances, with respect to socio-economic and health depreciation rates, to invest in different amounts of health. This is not to say that it will be optimal from a normative point of view. Equality in, say, utilization or health status might still be preferred by the policy-

---

[17] This should perhaps be classified as a certain type of *moral hazard*.

[18] In addition to the role as a perfect agent the physician often also have the role as representing the health care system with tasks such as *gate-keeping* or making rationing decisions.

[19] Although not easy to investigate empirically.

makers. However, it does put some restrictions on public health policy.[63] If the preferred principle is equal access to health care the Grossman model adds to the discussion about the relevant prices that affect people's behaviour. With respect to health behaviour it is not the price of health care per se that is important, even if transport costs and opportunity costs of spending time away from work were included in the price of health care. As the demand for health care is derived demand for health capital the relevant price is the unobserved shadow price of health capital. Although less tangible, one could imagine the health care system aiming to equalize the shadow prices of health capital[20]. This would require that the user costs of capital are the same for everyone or that the marginal costs of health investments, if counted on the supply side, are adjusted to offset differences in user costs of capital. That is, health care costs should be lower for people with higher depreciation rates. However, even for equal shadow prices, the investments in health, if people can choose freely, would differ across groups as the marginal efficiency of capital varies across groups. To obtain equality in health, the demand curve should also be adjusted, for example, by adjusting income or the human capital component. If equal health is the primary objective, the target of equal health status could be achieved for various levels of the shadow price by adjusting supply and/or demand for health capital to the appropriate level of health capital.

Personal preferences do also play a role in health behaviour. If the consumption aspect is sizeable compared to the investment aspect, it will be more difficult to determine the effect of different determinants as the consumption part of the model has less clear predictions.

In real life, the individual supply and demand curves as well as some of the determinants of these curves are not observable to the policy makers. However, the model does indicate some of the restrictions or consequences of some types of public health policies. Complete consumer sovereignty does not have to be assumed. The policy makers can control some of the variables such as the principles of allocation of health care services, e.g. equal treatment for equal need.

---

[20] It is still a normative question whether equal shadow prices of health capital are more equitable than equal prices of health care observed to everyone. In addition there are practical arguments for choosing one over the other.

But the policy makers can seldom control all of the relevant variables, and the uncontrollable variables have to be taken into account if unexpected outcomes are to be avoided.

Measuring distributional inequality or inequity

Operationalization of definitions
Given the multitude of definitions and interpretations of distributional justice it can be quite difficult to measure whether distributions of health and health care are in accordance with specific principles. The empirical literature has mainly focused on measuring inequality or certain distributional aspects that could indicate inequity given certain assumptions.

If the distributional principles to be used in the health care sector are different from the distributional principles that are used in the society in general then the distribution of other goods such as, for example, income or education, or the position in society in general, should not influence the distribution of health or health care (or perhaps only to a certain degree). Therefore, the distribution of health and health care are often characterized in relation to some socio-economic status variable.

With respect to health care the question is often whether actual utilization or access should be the focus of the analysis. As access, in the sense of opportunity to use, is a more intangible concept, the distributional analyses of health care are most often carried out as utilization studies,[16] and this is suggested by some researchers who are advocates of equal access.[47,82-85] This approach can be justified in the likelihood that inequality in access would lead to inequality in utilization (although equal utilization would not necessarily be guaranteed by equal access). Whether utilization or access is the focus, need is often taken into account as suggested by the egalitarian principles *equal treatment for equal need* or *equal access for equal need*. The various definitions of need can be difficult to operationalize, and health status and some socio-demographic characteristics are often used as proxies for need for health care.[86-89] As a consequence, when need is controlled for this way, the measures reduce to the horizontal variants of the egalitarian equity principles. The vertical variants can only be operationalized if it is specified how people in different need situations should be compensated with different levels of health care utilization or access.[90]

When the focus is on *equal health* there is no need to take need-based characteristics into account. However, if some health differences across socio-demographic groups are acceptable or unavoidable these characteristics can be taken into account in the description of the health distribution, and the measure becomes a horizontal variant of the equity principle.[91,92]

Measuring inequality

To characterize a distribution of health or health care with respect to how equal or unequal it is a quantitative measure is required. Different inequality measures measure different aspects of the inequality of a distribution. Pure equality characterizes a distribution when all the individuals in a population have the same amount of the variable of interest. Inequality then exists when the individuals have different amounts of the variable of interest. When the distribution is characterized in relation to some socio-economic variable, socio-economic equality exists when individuals from different socio-economic groups on average have a same amount of the variable of interest. Socio-economic inequality is present when individuals from some socio-economic groups on average have more of the variable of interest than individuals from other groups.

A measure tends to be called an index when it is normalized to a specified range, typically bounded by 0 and 1.[93] The measure is univariate if it characterizes the distribution of a single variable, i.e. pure inequality, and the measure is bivariate if it characterizes the distribution of a variable with respect to another variable, that is, socio-economic inequality.[94,95] A measure can be characterized with respect to whether it measures relative or absolute inequality. That is, whether the same relative growth for everyone will affect the size of the inequality measure. Furthermore, the inequality measure can include information for the entire population or compare only the most extreme groups or individuals. It is also important how and to what degree a transfer from one individual to another affects the size of the measure. Some measures are strictly descriptive, whereas others incorporate a certain social welfare function or include a parameter that reflects, for instance, inequality aversion.[96-101]

In addition, bivariate measures can be classified into measures of the effect of socio-economic status on the variable of interest, or into measures of the total impact of the distribution of the socio-economic variable on the variable of interest.[97]

According to Wagstaff et al., a measure of socio-economic inequality in health should minimally meet three requirements: 1) It should reflect the socio-economic dimension, 2) it should use information from the entire population, and 3) it should be sensitive to changes across individuals from different socio-economic groups.[100]

The concentration index

Among health economists the concentration index has become the standard measure for quantifying socio-economic inequality in health or health care.[1,85,88,89,91,92,99,102-109] The concentration index can be derived from the income inequality literature where the Gini coefficient has long been the traditional univariate inequality measure.[96,99] The concentration index is the bivariate generalization of the Gini coefficient and is a measure of how equal one variable is distributed with respect to the ranking of another variable[21].[110]

The concentration index can be illustrated graphically by the concentration curve. If the variable of interest is health and the socio-economic variable is income the concentration curve shows the cumulative share of health (the distribution function for health) as a function of the cumulative share of the population ranked by income (the fractional income-rank). An equal share of health across all income groups will make the concentration curve correspond to the diagonal.

If health is concentrated among the higher income-groups the concentration curve will be placed below the diagonal as in Figure 2a, and if health is concentrated among the lower income-groups the concentration curve will be situated above the diagonal as in Figure 2b.

---

[21] The Gini coefficient is a special case of the concentration index where the variable of interest is the same as the ranking variable. The graphical equivalent to the concentration curve is the Lorenz curve.

There are, of course, also situations where the curve will intersect the diagonal; for instance, if health is concentrated among the median income-groups as in Figure 2c[22]. A distribution is more unequal than another if its concentration curve is farther away from the diagonal than the other distribution's concentration curve (Figure 2d). However, if the curves intersect each other a summary measure is required to solve the matter.

The concentration curve can be summarized by the concentration index by measuring twice the area between the concentration curve and the diagonal with positive weight given to areas below the diagonal and negative weight given to areas above the diagonal. The concentration index C ranges between -1 and 1 and is positive if health is concentrated among the higher income-groups (Figure 2a), zero if there is complete equality or completely off-setting effects (Figure 2c)[23], and negative if health is concentrated among the lower income-groups (Figure 2b). C can be calculated as

$$C = \frac{2}{n\bar{y}} \sum_{i=1}^{n} y_i R_i - 1, \tag{8}$$

where y_i is the variable of interest, e.g. the health variable, $\bar{y}$ the mean of y_i, and R_i is the fractional rank, which is easily calculated as the unconditional rank with respect to income adjusted by 0.5 and divided by the sample population n [111]:

$$R_i = \frac{r - 0.5}{n}. \tag{9}$$

---

[22] The concentration curves for actual empirical distributions will, of course, take less smooth shapes than is shown in Figure 2.
[23] Whether perfectly off-setting effects are as good as perfect equality is a matter of opinion.

Figur 2. Examples of concentration curves

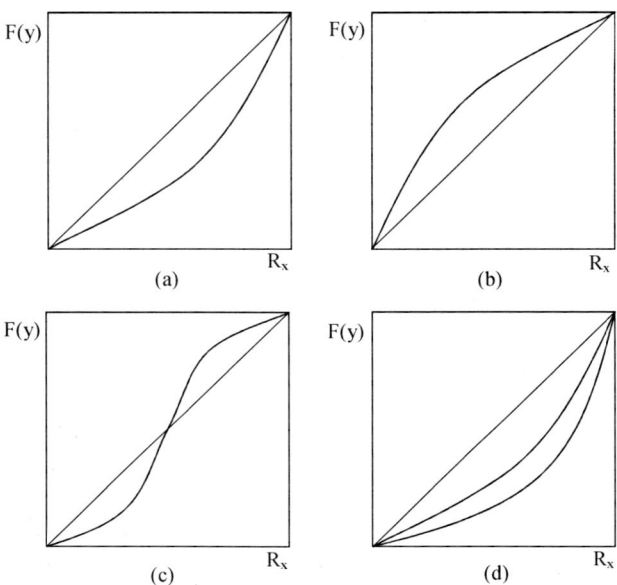

F(y) is the cumulative proportion of the variable y. R_x is the fractional rank of the variable x. (a) The variable y is concentrated among the higher percentiles of x. (b) The variable y is concentrated among the lower percentiles of x. (c) A concentration curve crossing the diagonal. The variable y is concentrated among the median percentiles of x. (d) Two convex concentration curves.

If weighted data are used, e.g. to adjust for stratified sampling procedures the health variable in (8) should be replaced by a weighted version: $y_{wi} = w_i y_i$ (and correspondingly $\bar{y}_w = \sum w_i y_i / n$), where w_i is the weight of individual i normalized so that $\sum w_i = n$. Using weighted data Lerman et al. have shown that the accuracy of the fractional rank can be improved by

$$R_i = \frac{1}{n}\sum_{j=1}^{n-1} w_j + 0.5 w_i, \qquad w_0 = 0, \tag{10}$$

where w_i is the individual's weight, and w_j the cumulative sum of weights.[112]

An easy way to estimate the concentration index is to use the so-called convenient regression where the relative health of the individual, multiplied by twice the variance of the fractional rank is regressed on the fractional rank:[110]

$$2\sigma_R^2 \frac{y_i}{\bar{y}} = \beta_0 + \beta_1 R_i + \varepsilon_i \ . \tag{11}$$

The OLS estimator for β_1 is equal to C, and this is the case whether or not the OLS assumptions are met. The standard error for β_1 is easily obtained from the regression for inference of the concentration index, although it should only be seen as an approximation as the errors in the regression may (or may not) be serially correlated.[110] Kakwani et al. have suggested a correction for this potential serial correlation[24].[111] However, this correction is not appropriate if weighted data are used.[113]

Properties of the concentration index

The concentration index fulfills the three minimal requirements suggested by Wagstaff et al.,[100] and it has other noteworthy characteristics.

    The concentration index includes a socio-economic dimension by having the ranking variable sorted by a socio-economic variable.

    The index is a measure of the total impact of socio-economic position (although it says nothing about causality). The concentration index uses information from the entire population, and not just the higher and lower socio-economic groups, although the inequality of the socio-economic variable is only reflected by the rank and not by the distributional characteristics of that variable. This way the index is not sensitive to changes in group sizes over time with regard to the

---

[24] Taking into account the serial correlation, the variance of C can be obtained by
$Var(C) = \frac{1}{n}\left[\frac{1}{n}\sum_{i=1}^{n} a_i^2 - (1+C)^2\right]$, where $a_i = \frac{y_i}{\bar{y}}(2R_i - 1 - C) + 2 - q_{i-1} - q_i$, and
$q_i = \frac{1}{\mu n}\sum_{\gamma=1}^{i} y_i$. q_i is the ith ordinate of the concentration curve.[111]

calculation of the index, although the (distribution of) group characteristics, as we shall see, can have an impact on the inequality.

The concentration index is sensitive to redistribution of health across groups.[114] If individual i receives an amount of health d from individual j such that individual i has $y_i + d$ and and j has $y_j - d$, then the change in C is

$$\Delta C = \frac{2}{n\overline{y}} d(R_i - R_j). \tag{12}$$

If individual i has a lower income than individual j then $R_i < R_j$ and ΔC is clearly negative and equivalent to less pro-rich inequality in health, no matter where on the income scale the two individuals are to be found. The size of the change in C depends on the relative ranks, that is, the share of the ranked population in between the two individuals. That is, it doesn't matter how much they already have, that is, the sizes of y_i and y_j are of no importance for the redistributive effect of d on C.[114]

The concentration index is also sensitive to a change in income ranks, for instance, if two individuals exchange income positions such that individual i increases his position with $R_j - R_i$ and individual j decreases his position with the same amount. Then the change in C is

$$\Delta C = \frac{2}{n\overline{y}} (R_j - R_i)(y_i - y_j). \tag{13}$$

If individual i has a lower income than individual j then $(R_j - R_i)$ is positive and the sign of ΔC depends on $(y_i - y_j)$. For a given distribution in health the size of the concentration index can be modified by redistributing health across income groups or changing the income rank[25].

The concentration index can be characterized, as the name suggests, as an index as it is bounded by -1 and 1. However, unlike a correlation coefficient the concentration index is also a function of the

---

[25] This is how the concentration index works. Whether this kind of redistribution or reranking is a desirable or practical way to meet some policy objectives is a different matter.

relative variation in y (the coefficient of variation)[26].[110] That is, for a constant correlation between the health variable and the ranking variable the concentration index will be bigger for a higher variability in health. It should also be noted that if the variable of interest is a dichotomous variable then the possible boundaries are numerically smaller than -1 and 1. Wagstaff has pointed out that the concentration index is bounded by approximately $\bar{y}$ - 1 and 1 - $\bar{y}$, That is, a higher mean diminishes the range of possible values and this should be taken into account when evaluating different dichotomous variables.[115]

The concentration index is a relative index.[116] Scaling up the health for everyone with the same percentage does not change the index[27]. Adding a constant to everyone's health does, however, change the index as the coefficient of variation is affected. According to Clarke et al., the consequence is that it does matter, for example, whether a health measure or an ill-health measure is used as a health status measure.[116] Typically, the variation in health relative to overall health status is much smaller compared to the variation in ill-health relative to the overall level of ill-health. An alternative specification, suggested by Clarke et al., is the generalized concentration index which is the concentration index multiplied by the mean of the variable of interest [116]:

$$C_{generalized} = \bar{y}C. \tag{14}$$

The generalized concentration index expresses the inequality in terms of the mean, and presents the same (numerical) index estimates if health and ill-health are complements of each other. However, the generalized concentration index is not bounded by -1 and 1 as $\bar{y}$ depends on the unit of measurement. The examination of these properties also leads to the

---

[26] Koolman et al. has shown that the concentration index can also be written as

$$C = \frac{\sigma_y}{\bar{y}} \rho(y, R) \frac{12\sigma_R^2}{\sqrt{3}}.$$ That is, C depends on the coefficient of variation, the correlation coefficient, and the variance of the rank multiplied by a constant.[110]

[27] Scaling up everyone's health variable, for instance, with a growth rate g in formula 8 results in $C_{1+g} = \frac{2}{n\sum_{i=1}^{n}(1+g)y_i} \sum_{i=1}^{n}(1+g)y_i R_i - 1 = \frac{(1+g)2}{(1+g)n\bar{y}} \sum_{i=1}^{n} y_i R_i - 1$, which keeps C in formula 8 unchanged.

question about what types of variables we can use for the concentration index. From a mathematical point of view the mean of y cannot be zero as this mean is used in the denominator of formula 8.[117] For the purpose of interpreting the concentration index the use of interval scale variables is problematic as C is sensitive to the choice of the zero point.[116] This means that the concentration index is appropriate only for ratio-scaled variables[28]. However, Allison has pointed out that valid comparisons can be made for interval scales (for Gini coefficients) if it is believed that the scales represent and underlying ratio-scale.[96] The underlying ratio scale implies a natural zero which limits the choice of the zero point for the interval scale. Chen et al. have looked into the problems of negative values of the variable of interest (for the Gini coefficient)[29].[118] When the variable of interest is negative the concentration curve can possibly intercept the upper or lower horizontal axes of the concentration curve diagram. Chen suggests that the diagram is expanded downwards (or upwards) to include the positive and negative part of the concentration curve, such that twice the area between the diagonal and the concentration index is compared to this expanded diagram.[118] The ranking variable for the concentration index has to be at least ordinal scaled, such that values of the ranking variable, as the name suggests, can be ranked.

Interpretation of the concentration index in terms of redistribution
As shown earlier, the concentration index has the useful property that it can be presented graphically. This facilitates an intuitive understanding of the concentration index. However, there is no easy intuitive interpretation of the size of the estimated concentration index. Koolman et al. have suggested a hypothetical linear redistribution scheme to assist an intuitive interpretation.[110] If formula 11 is used to estimate the concentration index we know that the least squares line goes though the means of the transformed health variable, $2\sigma_R^2 y_i/\bar{y}$, and the fractional

---

[28] Perhaps the exception is dichotomous variables as they also have natural zero points if zero-one coding is used.
[29] The problems of negative values for variables used for the concentration index have to some extent been ignored in the literature. For instance, variables with negative values have been used by Wagstaff et al. and by Zere et al.[85,117]

rank, r_i, which is $2\sigma_R^2$ and 0.5 (for unweighted data), respectively. If the slope of this line is zero the concentration index is also zero. A zero sloped line can be obtained by transferring transformed health (linearly) from the part of the line that is above the mean of $2\sigma_R^2 y_i/\bar{y}$ to the part that is below the mean by making each individual transfer $(R_i-0.5)\beta_1$ to an individual with fractional rank 1 - R_i. That is, half of $0.5(0.5)\beta_1$ needs to be transferred. As a share of aggregate transformed health this is $(1/8)\beta_1/(2\sigma_R^2)$ which can be reduced to $(3/4)\beta_1$ if it is taken into consideration that σ_R^2 is approximately equal to 1/12 for large samples. As y is related proportionally to $2\sigma_R^2 y_i/\bar{y}$ it means that aggregate health should be multiplied by $(3/4)C$ to find the amount of overall health that should be transferred linearly from the upper or lower 50 percentiles (of the ranking variable) where health is concentrated to the other 50 percentiles to reduce the concentration index to zero given a linear redistribution scheme. The linear redistribution scheme helps to interpret the size of a given concentration index estimate. However, this scheme is only one redistribution scheme among other potential designs.[110] One consequence of actually following this scheme would be the risk that health would be transferred from some individuals with low health status to some individuals with high health status as some variation in health is to be expected in both ends of the income scale. Some individuals can even end up with negative values. Furthermore, the transfers are, of course, only hypothetical if the variable of interest is health, as health cannot really be redistributed. However, health can be modified across individuals to a certain extent, and if the variable of interest is health care, then this variable can certainly be redistributed across individuals.

Inequality aversion in the concentration index

The concentration index can be thought of as a descriptive measure as it objectively measures the area between the concentration curve and the diagonal in a concentration curve diagram. However, Wagstaff has drawn attention to the fact that the concentration index is equivalent to an implicit weighting of the ranked observations, and that other weighting mechanisms are also possible.[119] Wagstaff has showed that formula 8 is a special case of a formula for the concentration index. The general case can be written as

$$C(\upsilon) = 1 - \frac{1}{n\bar{y}} \sum_{i=1}^{n} y_i \upsilon (1-R_i)^{\upsilon-1}, \qquad \upsilon \geq 1 \tag{15}$$

where υ is a parameter for how the different observations should be ranked. A value of υ higher than 1 denotes that lower ranked observations are weighted more than higher ranked observations. For a value of 2 the formula reduces to formula 8[30]. For higher values of υ progressively more weight is given to the lower ranked observations. The upper values of $C(\upsilon)$ are bound by 1 as in the special case of $\upsilon = 2$. However, in the general case the lower values can exceed -1, numerically, if the health variable is concentrated among the lower ranked individuals. The parameter υ can be used as an inequality aversion parameter with higher values representing more aversion to inequality[31].[119] However, the parameter says more about the kind of inequality we are measuring than the actual aversion to equality. The trade-off with other objectives is a separate issue. The attention to the fact that the concentration index is a special case of a more general formulation is important because it reminds us that the concentration index measures only a certain kind of inequality in the distribution that might or might not be in accordance with our preferred principles for equitable arrangements in the health care sector.

Alternative measures

The analysis above should also remind us that the concentration index is only one measure among many inequality measures. Other measures would have other properties or measure different aspects of equality of distributions.

---

[30] A value of $\upsilon = 2$ results in weights $(\upsilon(1-R_i)^{\upsilon-1})$ of approximately 2 for the lowest ranked observation and linearly decreasing weights over the range R_{min}-R_{max} with the highest ranked observation having a rank of approximately zero.

[31] Wagstaff suggested that formula 15 could be used in a social welfare function of the form: $SWF(\upsilon) = \bar{y}(1-C(\upsilon))$, where the size of the inequality aversion parameter υ would indicate the preferred trade-off between inequality and efficiency.[119]

If the focus is on pure inequality in health (or health care) an obvious choice would be the Gini-coefficient. As the Gini-coefficient is a special case of the concentration index, where the variable of interest is identical to the ranking variable, the properties are roughly the same. However, an analysis of transfers is a bit more complicated as the observations can possibly change ranking position due to the transfers.[110] Other possible measures of pure inequality include the range, the variance, the Pietra-ratio, the Theil index, and the Atkinson index[32]. The range measures the relative differences between the most extreme groups, but ignores the intermediate groups.[99,100] The measure is therefore insensitive to redistributions unless the most extreme groups are affected. The Pieatra-ratio (also called the Schutz coefficient or the Robin Hood index) measures the share of the health variable that needs to be transferred from above average individuals to below average individuals to obtain equality.[93,110] The index is sensitive to transfers, but only if they occur between individuals on each side of the mean. The measure does have a graphical interpretation in that the amount needed for the transfer is equal to the maximum vertical distance between the diagonal and the univariate concentration curve (Lorenz curve) in a concentration curve diagram. The variance is sensitive to redistributions on one side of the mean as deviations further from the mean are weighted higher. However, the variance depends on the mean level and is not normalized to 0 and 1.[99] The measure can be turned into a relative measure by relating it to the mean.[99] A common measure with this property is the coefficient of variation, CV, which is

---

[32] The formulas for pure inequality measures: The Gini coefficient:

$G = \frac{2}{n\bar{y}} \sum_{i=1}^{n} y_i R_{yi} - 1$; the range: $R = (Max(y_i) - Min(y_i))/\bar{y}$; The Pietra

Ratio: $S = \frac{1}{2n\bar{y}} \sum_{i=1}^{n} |y_i - \bar{y}|$; the variance: $\sigma^2 = \frac{1}{n} \sum_{i=1}^{n} (\bar{y} - y_i)^2$, and the $CV = \frac{\sigma}{\bar{y}}$;

Theil's entropy index: $T = \sum_{i=1}^{n} \left(\frac{y_i}{\bar{y}}\right) \ln\left(\frac{y_i}{\bar{y}}\right)$; Atkinson's index:

$A = 1 - \left[\frac{1}{n} \sum_{i=1}^{n} \left(\frac{y_i}{\bar{y}}\right)^{1-\varepsilon}\right]^{\frac{1}{1-\varepsilon}}$, $0 \leq \varepsilon \leq \infty$.

nevertheless not limited by 0 and 1. Another measure from the income inequality literature is Theil's measure of inequality.[93,96,110] The index satisfies the principle of transfers as redistribution from the better off to the worse off decreases the index value. However, as the upper limit of the index depends on the sample size, differentials between samples can be hard to interpret. The Atkinson measure takes inequality aversion into account by comparing social welfare generated by the actual distribution compared to social welfare for an equal distribution. Using a concave social welfare function the social welfare cannot become higher than an equal distribution, and this bounds the Atkinson measure between 0 and 1.[93,96,110]

If the focus is on socio-economic inequality in health (or health care) a number of alternatives to the concentration index has been used in the literature. Among the most common measures are the ratio, the index of dissimilarity, correlation and regression measures, and correlations with ranks[33]. A widely used measure is the ratio comparing the lowest with the highest socio-economic group, and this measure is often estimated as a rate-ratio or an odds-ratio in social epidemiology.[97,120] This measure includes only the most extreme groups and is insensitive to changes in the population not included in these groups. Furthermore, the estimated ratio will most likely depend on the cut-off points for the most extreme groups.[100] Another

---

[33] The formulas for bivariate inequality measures: The rate-ratio: $rr = \dfrac{\tau_{low}}{\tau_{high}}$; the index of dissimilarity: $ID = \dfrac{1}{2}\sum_{j=1}^{J}|P_{j,health} - P_{j,population}|$; correlation coefficient: $\rho = \dfrac{\sigma_{xy}}{\sigma_x \sigma_y}$; regression coefficient: $\hat{\beta}_1$ estimated from the regression $y_i = \beta_0 + \beta_1 x_i + \varepsilon_i$. The SII can be obtained by $\hat{\beta}_1$ from $y_i = \beta_0 + \beta_1 R_i + \varepsilon_i$, the RII can calculated as $\hat{\beta}_1 / \bar{y}$, or in another version as $(\hat{\beta}_0 - \hat{\beta}_1)/\hat{\beta}_0$, whereas the concentration index C is equal to $2\sigma_R^2 \hat{\beta}_1 / \bar{y}$.

measure is the index of dissimilarity which is based on the differences between health shares and population shares for the different socio-economic groups and should be interpreted as the percentage of health that has to be redistributed to obtain equality among the groups.[97,100,120,121] The order of the groups is not incorporated in the index such that the ranking of the groups is not reflected. However, for nominal variables for socio-economic status (e.g. occupational status) that might be a convenient feature. As socio-economic inequality in a health-related variable is a bivariate issue it is natural to use a measure of association such as a correlation coefficient or a regression coefficient for the association between the two variables. The appropriateness of these measures depends on whether the focus is on the correlation alone or on correlation and variation.[120] The variation is not included in measures of association.[110] Other measures, like the concentration index, use the fractional rank of the socio-economic variable. The most common of these measures are the relative index of inequality (RII) and the slope index of inequality (SII).[97,100,110,120,121] Both measures can be obtained by regressing the health variable on the fractional rank of the socio-economic variable. The RII presents the association in relative terms (like the concentration index) whereas the SII presents the association in natural units (like the generalized concentration index). The two measures suffer from the fact that they don't have the same graphical representation as the concentration index.

This section served the purpose of reminding us that there are alternatives to the concentration index when measuring the inequality of a distribution. Each measure has strengths and weaknesses and would potentially result in different rankings of comparable distributions. The appropriateness of applying the different measures depends on the type of inequality we want to measure.

Standardizing the concentration index

As was shown in the previous sections the concentration index measures how one variable (e.g. health or health care) is distributed with respect to the ranking of another variable (e.g. income).[110] The differences between the observations are compared to a baseline case of an equal distribution (the diagonal in the concentration index diagram). By using the concentration index it is not taken into consideration that some individuals, given the preferred principles for allocation of health or health care, are expected to have smaller or larger shares of the variable of interest.

If the focus is on health care, and we want to examine the egalitarian principle of *equal treatment for equal need*, then we ought to take into account that some of the differences in health care utilization are caused by differences in need. Need can be difficult to operationalize, and health status and some socio-demographic variables are often used as proxies for need.[87-89,122] If the focus is on *equal health* need as such is not relevant. However, even when measuring inequality in health it might be appropriate to take into consideration that individuals are different from each other, for instance, with respect to socio-demographic variables such age and gender. The socio-demographic variables can be taken into account by standardizing the concentration index with respect to these variables.

The necessity to standardize arises because only the horizontal variants of the egalitarian principles have been specified. Given the vertical variants of the principles we know that unequal people, with regard to certain specified characteristics, should be in correspondingly unequal conditions or treated unequally. However, we don't know how much, as the vertical variants of the principles have not been operationalized. The standardization removes the inequality due to the standardizing variable such that the mean level of the variable of interest, y_i, given the various levels of standardizing variables, is seen as a measure for the appropriate level. The horizontal variant can then be seen as equality given a level of the standardizing variables. That is, people are practically compared to people with the same levels of the standardizing variables.

Gravelle et al. have discussed the conditions for treating variables as standardizing variables.[90,91,123] Whether a variable should be treated as a standardizing variable depends on the circumstances. To Gravelle, a variable should be used to standardize if it is impossible to alter its effect on the variable of interest or its joint distribution with the ranking variable. This is also a question of policy context as some variables might be perceived as given in some situations and perceived as changeable in other situations.[52,91]

There are several ways to standardize the concentration index. An indirect method of standardization is to compare the concentration curve with a concentration curve for the new expected baseline level given the standardizing variables.[1,88] The expected level given the standardizing variables can be estimated by the regression:

$$y_i = \beta_0 + \sum_Z \beta_Z x_{Zi} + \varepsilon_i,\qquad(16)$$

where the x_{zi}s are the standardizing variables. The average level given the standardizing variables can be estimated for each observation by

$$y_i^* = \hat{\beta}_0 + \sum_Z \hat{\beta}_Z x_{Zi},\qquad(17)$$

and a standardized concentration index, I, can be calculated as

$$I = C - C^*,\qquad(18)$$

where C^* is the concentration index estimated for the y_i^*s. Applied on health care this measure is also called the index of horizontal inequity, HI, as it evaluates the principle of *equal treatment for equal need*.[1,88] This index can, in the most extreme cases, vary between -2 and 2, as all the health care could be given to the lowest ranked observation, and if, at the same time, the highest ranked observation would be the only one in need, or vice versa. The standard error for I is not easily obtained as C and C^* are not independently distributed.[88,111] However, the standard error and the standardized concentration index can be obtained from the convenient regression by including $y_i^*/\bar{y}^*$ in addition to $y_i/\bar{y}$ on the left-hand side of the regression from formula 11:

$$2\sigma_R^2 \left[\frac{y_i}{\bar{y}} - \frac{y_i^*}{\bar{y}^*} \right] = \beta_0 + \beta_1 R_i + \varepsilon_i.\qquad(19)$$

The estimated β_1 is equal to the standardized concentration index.[88] As mentioned above, the standard error from the convenient regression should only be seen as an approximation as the errors may be serially correlated.

The problem with formula 16 is that it might suffer from omitted variable bias.[91] A standardizing variable might be correlated with the ranking variable, say income, such that part of the influence of the standardizing variable on y_i is due to variations in income. In addition, other variables could be correlated with y_i for given level of income. To control for those variables, they can be included in the standardizing regression:

$$y_i = \beta_0 + \beta_1 x_{Ii} + \sum_Z \beta_Z x_{Zi} + \sum_S \beta_S x_{Si} + \varepsilon_i , \qquad (20)$$

where x_{Ii} is income and the x_{Si}s are other explanatory variables. To obtain the effect of the standardizing variables, without the effect of the other variable, the y_i^*s can be predicted by formula 20 by neutralizing the effect by the other variables by setting them to their means.[124]

$$y_i^* = \hat{\beta}_0 + \hat{\beta}_1 \bar{x}_{Ii} + \sum_Z \hat{\beta}_Z x_{Zi} + \sum_S \hat{\beta}_S \bar{x}_{Si} . \qquad (21)$$

If y_i is only correlated with the standardizing variables then formula 17 works for non-linear regression functions as well ($y_i = f(\sum x_{zi})$). However, a non-linear specification for relations such as formula 21 is problematic as the effect of the standardizing variables depends on the levels chosen for the non-standardizing variables, such as the means – as chosen for this equation. Therefore, the other variables cannot be expected to be completely neutralized.[124] An alternative approach is to use a linear approximation of the marginal effects of the regression in formula 21 in a decomposition framework. The decomposition approach to standardization is what Gravelle calls direct standardization[34].[91] Wagstaff et al. showed that if y_i is explained linearly by a number of explanatory variables such as x_{Ii}, $\sum x_{zi}$, and $\sum x_{si}$ from formula 20 then the concentration index can be written as a weighted sum of the concentration indices for the different explanatory variables (with respect to the ranking variable, say income) and weighted by their elasticities evaluated around their means [117]:

$$C = \frac{\beta_1 \bar{x}_1}{\bar{y}} C_I + \sum_Z \frac{\beta_Z \bar{x}_Z}{\bar{y}} C_Z + \sum_S \frac{\beta_S \bar{x}_S}{\bar{y}} C_S + \frac{1}{\bar{y}} CG_\varepsilon , \qquad (22)$$

The last term, $CG_\varepsilon/\bar{y}$ is a residual component and reflects the socio-economic inequality in y_i that cannot be explained by the explanatory variables.[117] The term is called the generalized concentration index but should not be confused with the generalized concentration index from formula 14. Formula 22 shows that an explanatory variable contributes to socio-economic inequality in y_i if the variable is unevenly

---

[34] In other settings direct standardization has referred to situations where the ranking variable has been grouped and each group adjusted to the same level of the standardized variables.

distributed across the socio-economic (ranking) variable, and if the explanatory variable is correlated with y_i. The standardized concentration index can be estimated as the sum of all the components from the non-standardizing variables, or to simplify things, as the observed concentration index minus the standardizing components [91,92,124]:

$$I = C - \sum_z \frac{\beta_z \bar{x}_z}{\bar{y}} C_z \qquad (23)$$

The question is whether the generalized concentration index should be counted as a standardizing or non-standardizing component. The residual term could be attributed to unexplained inequality or to unobserved need or acceptable differences.[124] If all relevant variables are included in the regression in formula 20 then the ranking variable and the error term should be uncorrelated. According to Gravelle the two approaches are asymptotically equivalent.[91] Furthermore, when the relation in formula 20 is linear then the indirect and direct standardization lead to the same results.[124]

The decomposition is based on OLS regression.[117] If the relation in formula 20 is non-linear then one solution is to approximate linear marginal effects in formula 22 from a non-linear regression.[124] Another solution is to approximate a linear relationship for the non-linear relationship with a linear regression.[89,105,125]

Given the discussion of the conditions for treating variables as standardizing variables formula 22 is convenient because if all the components of the decomposition are presented in a disaggregated form the reader can choose for himself whether the separated components should be counted as standardizing or non-standardizing components.[92]

Material and setting

Setting

The Danish health care system

To analyze the distribution of health and health care in the present studies a combination of survey data and register-based data has been used. The data cover individuals living in Funen County, Denmark, during the years 2000 and 2001, and include information about health status and certain types of health care utilization. Funen County was, at the time of data collection, one county among 15 geographical units in Denmark (14 counties and the Copenhagen Hospital Corporation).[126-128]

The institutional characteristics of the health care system can possibly play a role in the distribution of health and health care.[88,89,92,124] The Danish health care system, as it was around the time of data collection, is therefore briefly described in the following section. The Danish health care system is a decentralized multi-level single-payer system with comprehensive and universal coverage, and it is financed mainly through the general tax system, particularly by county taxes.[126-128] The system was, at the time of data collection, organized into three levels: the state level, the county level, and the municipal level. At state level the government prepared legislation and provided guidelines and supervision of the health care system. In addition, the government negotiated with the county councils about targets for the growth of health care expenditures.[127] The financing, priority setting and planning of the health care sector were delegated to the county level. The counties, with directly elected county councils, owned and ran the hospitals. Furthermore, the counties ran the National Health Security System which finances private practitioners in the primary health care sector such as general practitioners (GPs), practising specialists, dentists, physiotherapists, and reimbursements for prescription medicine. The county expenditures were financed by proportional county income taxes and real estate taxes (87%) and state grants (13%).[126-128] The municipalities, with directly elected municipal councils, financed and ran nursing homes, home nursing, and school health services, including the municipal school dentistry.[127]

Universal coverage exists so that health care services are free (or almost free) at the point of delivery. However, the GPs have a special role in the Danish health care system. They act as *gate keepers*, such that referral from the GP is necessary for treatment elsewhere in the health care system at the expense of the public sector[35]. Acute care and care by certain specialties, e.g. ear, nose and throat, are exempt from referral by the GP, and can be accessed free of charge without referral.[127,129]

For some types of health care a considerable degree of co-payment is present. In 2001, co-payment constituted 18-19 percent of the overall health expenditures.[129] Consultations at the GP, visits at the hospital (including medicine given at the hospital) and specialist treatment after referral were for free at the point of use. For dentistry, physiotherapy, and medicine the co-payment may be considerable. For dentistry for adults the size of the co-payment was attributable to the specific service and varied between 35 and 100 percent. The resulting average co-payment was close to 80 percent.[129] For physiotherapy the co-payment was the same percentage for all the services, 61 percent, although some patients were exempt from co-payment (The resulting co-payment was around 40 percent), whereas for prescription medicine the co-payment followed the individual at a decreasing rate such that large-scale consumers of medicine faced a lower percentage of co-payment. For the first DKK 500 (DKK 465 in 2007) of prescription medicine per year the co-payment constituted 100 percent of the price. The resulting average co-payment was close to one third of the prescription expenditures in 2001[36]. The reimbursement system for prescription medicine replaced a system of proportional subsidies in the spring of 2000.

Besides the National Health Security System, private insurance exists in Denmark. Around 30 percent of the population is

---

[35] 98 percent of the population belongs to this scheme (Group 1). People are free to choose a different scheme (Group 2) where referral to a specialist is not mandatory but involve considerable user-charges. Less than 2 percent has chosen this option.[127]
[36] From analyses carried out by Gundgaard et al.[130]

insured against co-payment by a non-profit organization known as *danmark*.[129] Furthermore, commercial insurance is becoming increasingly common for firms that offer insurance policies that include elective surgery and specialist treatment for their employees.[129] However, at the time of data collection these private health insurance schemes were only prevalent to a limited degree.[127] Private hospitals do exist but constitute less than 1 percent of all hospitals in terms of somatic hospital beds.[129] The extent to which private practitioners work privately, outside the scope of the National Health Security System, is not well known.

As of January 2007, a reform changed the structure of the Danish health care system. The system is kept as a multi-level system with three levels. However, the 15 counties have been reduced to 5 regions, and small municipalities have been merged into larger municipalities with increased responsibility for prevention and public health initiatives. The regions are partly financed by needs-adjusted state block grants (80 percent) from a national earmarked proportional health tax, and by reimbursements from municipalities (20 percent). The purpose of the reform is for the central government to get more control with regional and municipal levels and to improve the co-operation between the organizational levels (regions and municipalities).[126,128] The general arrangements with respect to coverage and co-payment have not been changed with the implementation of the reform.

Objectives of the Danish health care system

According to Pedersen et al., there has been no coherent and official statement of the goals of the Danish health care system. However, various objectives can be deduced from laws and government documents.[129] In the law of the health care sector from 2005 it was stated that the objective of the health care sector is to improve public health and to treat and prevent disease, suffering, and limitations in functioning. Furthermore, the health care sector is required to secure the respect for the individual, its integrity, its right of self-determination, and to fulfill the requirements of 1) free and equal access to the health care sector; 2) high quality treatment; 3) coherent services; 4) choice; 5) access to information; 6) a transparent health care sector; and 7) short waiting time for treatment.[131] By these statements, the objective can be interpreted as a mix of efficiency, autonomy, and equity in the sense of procedural justice. However, this list of objectives is by no means exhaustive. Equity considerations are an integrated part of the Danish culture, and this has played a major role in a number of areas.[128] In two government documents on public health from 1999 and 2002 (by different governments) the concern for social inequalities in health has been stressed.[132,133] Both documents focus particularly on life-style determinants for inequality in health for marginalized groups such as differences in life-style with regard to tobacco, alcohol, diet and exercise.[134] The former also focuses on differences in working and living conditions, whereas the latter focuses more on individual responsibility.[132,133] To Pedersen et al., other objectives are present too in the Danish health care system, for instance geographical equality and cost containment, although this is not necessarily explicitly stated.[129]

Funen County

Funen County was one of the 15 geographical units until the reform in January 2007 where it was merged with other counties into the Region of Southern Denmark. Situated in the middle of Denmark Funen County consisted of the islands of *Fyn*, *Ærø*, and *Langeland*, and about 90 other small islands. The county population made up a little less than 10 percent of the Danish population, or 472,100 inhabitants at the end of 2000.[135] The county was divided into 32 municipalities with Odense, the county capital, being the biggest (183,700 inhabitants at the end of 2000).[135] At the time of data collection the Funen hospital sector consisted of 9 hospitals divided into two hospital corporations with Odense University Hospital as the biggest one. Funen County was representative for Denmark in many respects. Table 1 compares Funen County with the national level with respect to some key figures regarding health care expenditures, consultations in the primary health care sector, and socio-demographic structure. As can be seen in the table, Funen County was fairly similar to the rest of the country.

In the year 2000, the county council released a document on the prevention strategy for improvement of public health in Funen County.[137] The strategy was inspired by the government document from 1999 but adjusted to local settings.[133,137] The overall

Table 1. Funen County compared to national data from the year 2000

	Expenditures per capita, DKK[†]		Contacts per 1000[†]				Mean age[‡]	
	Hospital	Primary care	GP	Specialist	Dentist		Men	Women
Funen County	8209	2426	6041	760	1067		37.9	40.4
Denmark	8296	2462	6086	866	1030		37.3	39.8

[†]The Ministry of Interior and Health,[136] Statbank Denmark, BEF1
[‡]Statbank Denmark, BEF1.[135]
[†]Expenditures given in 2000 price level.

objectives were stated as more life-years with a higher quality of life, and a reduction in social inequality in health, in particularly by improving health for the worst-off groups. In addition, there were some intermediate aims of improving health behaviour, with a specific focus on tobacco use, alcohol consumption, diet, and exercise. A number of preventive initiatives were put into action, and to monitor the health status and health behaviour of the residents in Funen County a health survey was carried out by Gundgaard et al.[138] The health survey was planned to be repeated twice over the course of the ten years prevention plan to monitor the population over time. However, due to the health care reform, the monitoring of the Funen population was put to an end after the first health survey. The data from this survey constitute the foundation for the empirical analyses in this thesis. For this purpose the survey data were merged with register based data to obtain information on health care utilization.

The data set

Survey data

The Funen County Health Survey is a cross-sectional sample of the population of residents in Funen County in the age interval 16-80 (both years included).[138] The sample consists of 5,000 individuals drawn from the parent population of 362,132 individuals in the relevant age category.[135] The sample was stratified with respect to municipalities to make sure that large and small municipalities are represented. About three percent of the population in small municipalities (with less than 7,000 residents) has been sampled, whereas about one percent of the population in bigger municipalities (with more than 7,000 residents) has been sampled. Within the municipalities the individuals were randomly selected. The sample was drawn from the Centralised Civil Register for all residents with a permanent postal address in the beginning of September 2000 (people with name protection and people registered as exempt from research projects were excluded from the parent population). The sampled individuals were interviewed over the phone by interviewers from the Danish National Institute of Social Research in the period from October 2000 through April 2001, and were asked about their health status (EQ-5D and SF-36), health behaviour (including smoking, alcohol, diet, and exercise), and socio-economic status (including income, education, and occupation).[138]

Due to non-response (and oversampling) not all individuals from the sample participated in the survey. Non-response can have many causes, and the non-respondents have been classified into different types of non-response. The following categories were used: *Interviewed*, *Item non-response*, *Non-contacts*, *Refusals*, and a residual category of *Other*. People living outside Funen County or registered as dead at the time of data collection were regarded as not belonging to the parent population under investigation (i.e. oversampling), and were excluded from the analyses.[139] For the present study the category of item non-response contained missing observations due to failure of answering questions regarding income and health status, and dichotomous variables regarding life-style. For other (categorical) variables the item non-response was given a separate category and could therefore be included in the study.

Figure 3 shows the classification of drop-outs of the initial sample of 5,000 people, and Table 2 shows the number of individuals and the aggregate number of individuals in the different categories of non-response. The response-rate due to unit non-response (external non-response) is 69 percent. However, due to item non-response of about 10 percentage points (internal non-response), the overall response rate is 58 percent[37]. Especially the income question has been skipped by many respondents. Refusal is the biggest cause of non-response. Two thirds of the external non-response is caused by people refusing to participate. Only a small number of people has not been found and could therefore not be invited to the interview. Up to 18 calls have been made to get in touch with people.

In Table 3 the response rate and the proportion of non-respondents in each category of non-response are listed. The response and non-response rates are shown for different socio-demographic variables. Men have a higher response-rate than women, which is not in accordance with the literature.[140-144] However, the bigger non-response rate for women is partly caused by a high rate of item non-

---

[37] The internal non-response rate varies from article to article as different variables are used for different analyses.

Figure 3. Classification of drop-outs of the Funen County Health Survey

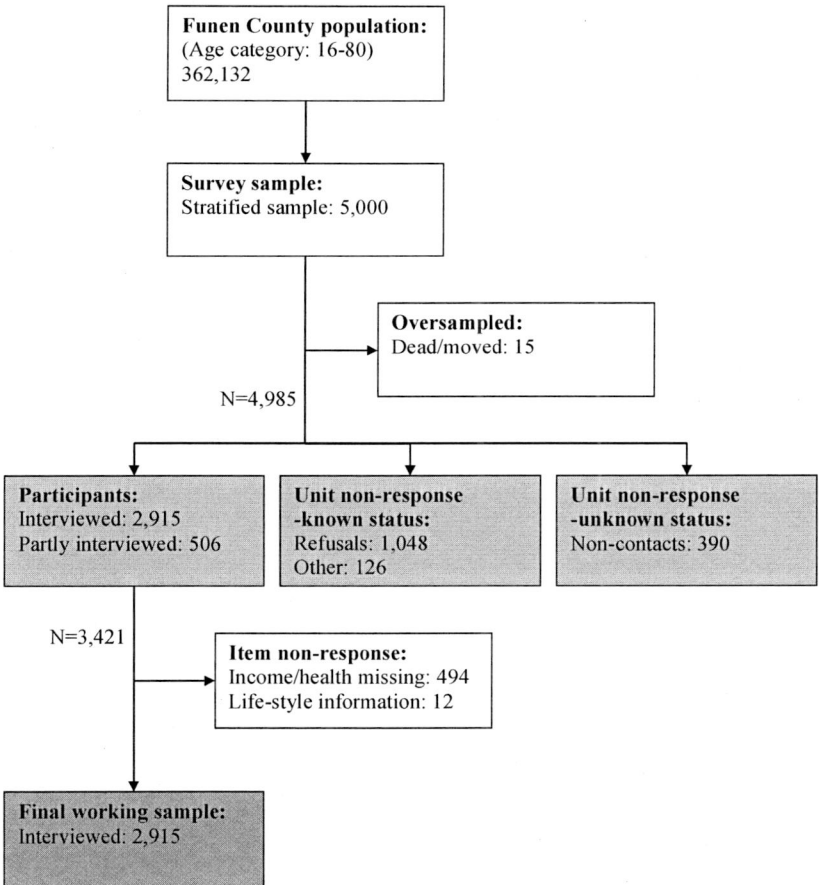

Notes: Nonresponse rate due to unit-nonresponse: (Interviewed + Item non-response)/(Interviewed + Item non-response + Non-contacts + other + refusals). Nonresponse rate due to unit-nonresponse and item-nonresponse: Interviewed/(Interviewed + Item non-response + Non-contacts + other + refusals). The figure is inspired by a report from the Section for Survey Statistics and Swedish Statistician Society.[139]

response. The age categories show the expected inverse u-formed relation with participation;[140,141,143,145,146] and among the marital status categories married people have a higher response rate than the rest of the categories. A thorough non-response analysis of the consequences for health care utilization estimates is presented in Chapter 7.

Register based data

The Funen County Health Survey was linked to individual-level computerized registers from various sources with information in health care utilization such as somatic hospital contacts, visits in the primary health care sector, and prescription medicine in 2000 and 2001.

The hospital visits were extracted from the Funen County Patient Administrative Database (FPAS), which includes records on all somatic inpatient stays, ambulatory and emergency room visits, and inspections from Odense University Hospital (including Middelfart) and the Sygehus Fyn hospital corporation (including hospitals in Bogense, Faaborg, Rudkøbing, Nyborg, Ringe, Svendborg, and Ærøskøbing)[38]. Each hospital admission is described by dates of admission/discharge, length of stay, diagnoses, DRG-group and DRG-charge.[147]

The data records on visits in the primary health care sector were extracted from the National Health Insurance Service Registry (National Health Security System) and delivered by the National Board of Health. This registry includes all partly or fully reimbursed health services in the primary health care sector. The services have been classified into treatment by general practitioners, specialists, physiotherapists, and dentists. A residual category of other services, including chiropractic, interpreters, some laboratory services, etc. was excluded from the analyses due to the heterogeneity and insignificance of these services. The records contain information on specialty, code for the service, subsidy from the National Health Security System, and the year for the service. More precise time for the service can be obtained but was not available for this study.

---

[38] The hospitals in Bogense and Rudkøbing have since then been shut down.

Table 2. Classification of respondents and non-respondents

		Detailed		Aggregated	
		n	percent	n	percent
interviewed	Participating	2915	58.48	2915	58.48
Item non-response	Income missing	483	9.69	506	10.15
	Health status missing	9	0.18		
	Income and health status missing	2	0.04		
	Life-style information missing	12	0.24		
Non-contacts	Gone away or in hospital	56	1.12	390	7.82
	Not contacted	273	5.48		
	Moved	49	0.98		
	No telephone	12	0.24		
Refusals	Refusal	995	20.00	1048	21.02
	Refusal and cannot be contacted again	53	1.06		
Other	Illness	37	0.74	126	2.53
	Handicapped	29	0.58		
	Other, including language problems	60	1.20		
Dead/moved	Live outside Funen	3	.	.	.
	Moved outside Denmark	6	.	.	.
	Dead	6	.	.	.

Table 2. (Continued) Notes:

N=4985 (Initial sample of 5000, 15 (Dead/moved) excluded from the analysis). Non-response rate due to unit-non-response ((Interviewed + Item non-response)/(Interviewed + Item non-response + Non-contacts + Other + refusals)): 68.63%. Nonresponse rate due to unit-nonresponse and item-nonresponse (Interviewed/(Interviewed + Item non-response + Non-contacts + Other + Refusals)): 58.48%.

Table 3. Proportion of respondents and non-respondents by socio-demographic variables

	Percent					Number	
	Interviewed	Item non-response	Non-contacts	Refusals	Other	$n_{interviewed}$	N_{all}
Total	58	10	08	21	3	2915	4985
Men	60	7	10	22	2	1476	2480
Women	57	14	06	20	3	1439	2505
16-24 years of age	55	13	16	14	2	340	621
25-44 years of age	63	08	9	18	2	1152	1841
45-66 years of age	60	09	6	23	2	1111	1850
67-80 years of age	46	15	3	30	5	312	673
Married	62	10	4	21	2	1650	2648
Not married	55	10	14	18	3	896	1621
Divorced	55	7	10	25	3	228	415
Widowed	47	11	4	34	3	141	301

Notes: N=4985 (Initial sample of 5000, 15 (Dead/moved) excluded from the analysis). See Table 2 for explanations for the different types of non-response.

Information on use of medicine was obtained from the Odense University Pharmacoepidemiologic Database (OPED).[148,149] This database consists of all prescription refunds from Funen County with partial or complete reimbursement. Prescription medicine not entitled to reimbursement (oral contraceptives, benzodiazepines, and certain antibiotics) and over-the-counter medicine (unless prescribed by the GP) are not included in the database.[149] Only pharmaceutical specialties are used for the analyses. Medicine used at hospitals is included in the hospital charges. The prescription records are described by date for purchase, sales number and name, quantity, ATC-code, Defined Daily Dose (DDD), and pharmacy retail price. The register based data have been validated against official statistics, and the agreement between the sources appeared to be good.[136,150-152]

Health care variables

For analyses concerning the distribution of health care, fees, charges, and retail prices have been used to operationalize health care utilization. This operationalization is expressed in variables for utilization of hospital treatment, GP services, specialist visits, physiotherapy, dental services, and utilization of prescription medicine. In addition, an aggregated variable has been created of all the different types of health care utilization added together. By using fees, charges, and retail prices the health care services are been measured in monetary terms. The advantage of using a common unit of measurement is that different types of services can be added together. Furthermore, the different services are weighted by the importance: a visit is not just a visit. Check-ups, for example, are weighted less than surgical treatments. Using information from registers made it possible to obtain exact information about the health care services for a long period of time (two years) without recall-bias. The registers also made it possible to distinguish between types of health care that have normally not been included in previous studies such as physiotherapy and prescription medicine.

Hospital contacts were described by estimated charges based on the 2002 Danish case mix system of Diagnosis Related Groups (DRGs). The case-mix system covers inpatient hospital stays, whereas ambulatory and emergency room visits are described by a similar but a more simple system. Inspections (of patients from other hospital departments) have not been given a charge. Furthermore, capital costs are not included in the case-mix system. All charges were adjusted to 2003 price level by the index for hospital treatments.[153]

For health care utilization in the primary health care sector each service is described by a reimbursement fee. As considerable co-payment exists for dental care and the physiotherapy the fees for these services have been adjusted to calculate the total amounts (reimbursement + co-payment). Expert judgments were used to adjust the fees for dental care to the average level of Funen dental care fees, whereas the relevant physiotherapist fees where adjusted by dividing the reimbursement fees with the proportion of reimbursement. All reimbursement fees were inflation adjusted to 2003 by the price index for physician and physiotherapist services.[153] General practitioners are partly financed through capitation (about one third of GP income). The GP fees have been adjusted for capitation in some analyses but not in other analyses.

The prescription records are described by pharmacy retail prices from the time of purchase including value-added tax. Some records with missing prices were given the latest available price. The pharmacy retail prices were inflation adjusted to 2003 level by the index for pharmaceutical products and equipment[39].[153]

An overview of the variables used in the study can be found in Table 4. Descriptive statistics of health care utilization across socio-demographic and socio-economic groups are presented in the Tables A1-A7 in the appendix to the chapter.

Health variables

Health variables are used for analyses regarding the distribution of health. To operationalize health, two health-related quality of life (HRQoL) measures have been used: EQ-5D and SF-36. The HRQoL measures were obtained from the Funen County Health Survey.[138]

---

[39] In one analysis the general CPI was used to inflation adjust the pharmacy retail prices.

The EQ-5D system is a standardized generic health instrument consisting of five dimensions of health: mobility, self-care, usual activities, pain/discomfort, and anxiety/depression.[154-156] Each dimension is divided into three levels of health: no problems, some or moderate problems, or extreme problems. The dimensions have been summarized into a single health index by weighting the levels of the dimensions by a standard set of general population preference time trade-off (TTO) weights established by Wittrup-Jensen et al[40].[159,160]

The SF-36 system is a widely used HRQoL measure of health status.[161-163] The SF-36 consists of 36 health questions that can be summarized by 8 scales for different dimensions of health: physical functioning, role-physical, bodily pain, general health perception, vitality, social functioning, role-emotion, and mental health. The 8 scales can further be summarized into two summary scores, PCS and MCS, for overall physical and mental health, respectively. The PCS and MCS were each calculated by standardizing each of the eight dimensions from the Danish SF-36, multiplying each dimension by its respective factor score coefficient, summing and standardizing to the American norm as recommended in Ware et al. and Bjørner et al.[164,165]

Descriptive statistics of EQ-5D TTO-value and the PCS and MCS scores across socio-demographic and socio-economic groups can be found in the Tables A8-A9 in the appendix.

Standardizing variables

For analyses of the distribution of health care the variables age, gender, and health status have been chosen as indicators of need. Age and gender are naturally given and not easy modifiable, although characteristics related to age and gender can be modified to some degree. Health status should only be seen as a proxy for need, although the use of health status is roughly in accordance with the *severity of illness* principle. Age has been included as a continuous variable in

---

[40] In some cases these values are called utilities, although certain assumptions have to be met for this to be true (in the von Neumann-Morgenstern sense of the word).[157,158] In this thesis the values are only perceived as a HRQoL index (a utility is not a utility is not a utility).[28]

some analyses and as age dummies in other analyses. Gender has been included as a dummy variable. Health status is represented by the EQ-5D TTO-value in some analyses and by a self-reported 5 categories health variable in other analyses (the first question in the SF-36 questionnaire).[164]

For analyses of the distribution of health no standardization has taken place. However, by using the decomposition method of standardization the reader can choose the standardization variables himself.

Socio-economic variables

The choice of socio-economic status variable depends on the purpose of the analysis. Income, education and occupation have been suggested as variables for socio-economic status.[166] For the present analysis income has been chosen as the ranking variable, as income is directly related to material conditions that may influence health and ability to pay for health care if access is limited. This choice of ranking variable narrows the present analyses to a focus on income-related inequality in health and health care.

Income is measured by self-reported gross income (gross of taxes and deductibles) from the previous year (1999) obtained from the Funen County Health Survey, and descriptive statistics have been validated against gross income from register based data. Income is a categorical variable consisting of 17 intervals. As a ranking variable the sample population is ranked according to the order of the categories. Within each category the respondents are ordered randomly. Income has also been used as an explanatory socio-economic variable, and the midpoint of the intervals were used to approximate a continuous income variable.

Education, occupation, and marital status are treated as other explanatory socio-economic variables. These variables are categorical variables – each with a category of *other* which includes, among other things, item non-response.

Table 4. Variables used in the study

	Variable	Explanation
Survey-based data:		
Health	EQ-5D	Danish TTO-value based on five dimensions: mobility, self-care, usual activities, pain/discomfort, anxiety/depression.
	SF-36	Summary scores: PCS (Physical Component Score), MCS (Mental Component Score) based on eight subscales: physical functioning, role-physical, bodily pain, general health perception, vitality, social functioning, role-emotion, mental health.
	SAH	Self-assessed health: 5 categories of general health (first question from the SF-36 questionnaire).
Socio-demo	Gender	Dummy variable: Men/Women.
	Age	Actual age or age dummy vector: 16-30, 31-45, 46-60, 61-70, 71-80.
Socio-econ	Income	Gross income in 1999 (gross of tax and deductibles). Midpoints of DKK income categories: <50000, 50000-99000, 100000-149000,…, >=749000.
	Education	Highest achieved education of primary, secondary, and tertiary education or vocational training. Classified into: Low education, Medium education High education, Other education (including item-non-response).
	Occupation	Regular occupation classified into: Unskilled, Skilled worker, White-collar, Selfemployed, Assisting spouse, Housewife, Student, Apprentice, Unemployed, Retired, Other occupation (including item non-response).
	Marital status	Marital status classified into: Married (including registered partnership), Cohabitant, Alone, Divorced, Separated, Widowed, Other status (including item non-response).

Table 4. (continued)

Life-style	Daily smoker	Dummy variably for daily smoking.
	High alcohol	Dummy variable for high alcohol intake: cut-off point at more than 21/14 units of alcohol per week for men/women.
	Vegetables, cooked	Dummy variable for eating cooked vegetables every day.
	Vegetables, raw	Dummy variable for eating raw vegetables every day.
	Fruit	Dummy variable for eating fruit every day.
	No exercises	Self-reported sedentary life-style.

Register-based data:

Health care	Hospital	Somatic hospital contacts 2000-2001, DRG-charges, DKK.
	GP	Services at the general practitioner 2000-2001, fees, DKK.
	Physiotherapy	Services at the physiotherapist 2000-2001, fees+co-payment, DKK.
	Specialist	Services at the specialist practitioner 2000-2001, fees, DKK.
	Dentist	Services at the dentist 2000-2001, fees or prices, DKK.
	Medicine	Prescription medicine with partial or complete reimbursement, pharmacy retail prices, DKK.
	Aggregate	Sum of all health care variables, DKK.

Life-style variables

Health-related life-style is represented by variables on smoking, alcohol, diet, and exercise. Due to the difficulties of reporting behaviour in this area the original variables from the Funen County Health Survey have been modified somewhat. Cut-off points have been used to classify the behaviour in dichotomous variables.[138]

The smoking variable is a binary variable for daily smoking. High alcohol consumption is a binary variable for a higher intake of alcohol than the recommended maximum of 21 and 14 units of alcohol per week for men and women, respectively. The dietary variables are binary variables for eating cooked vegetables, raw vegetables, and fruit, respectively, every day. The exercise variable is a binary variable for self-reported sedentary life-style.

Descriptive statistics of health-related life-style variables across socio-demographic and socio-economic groups can be found in Table A10 in the appendix.

Study design

The study design is a cross-sectional study design. The people participating have been interviewed only one time (in the period from October 2000 through April 2001) when they were asked about health status, health behaviour, and socio-economic characteristics. Health care has been measured over the course of two years (2000 and 2001) but is used in this cross-sectional study design as a point estimate of the flow of health care services over a period.

Given the cross-sectional study design we cannot be completely sure of the direction of causality. It is possible that there is some simultaneity in the relationship between health and health care or with other explanatory variables. As the study involves several potentially endogenous variables it would be difficult to deal with endogeneity of all variables, and the potential endogeneity is not accounted for. Therefore, relationships between variables represent statistical associations rather than causal effects and causal interpretations should be done with caution.

Guide to the empirical analyses

The empirical results are presented in Chapters 2 through 7. The chapters contain three analyses about the distribution of health care, two analyses about the distribution of health, and one analysis about the consequences of non-response for health care utilization estimates. The chapters reflect, to some degree, a progression over the three years work on the topic. The use of methods has been refined over the period, although the varying use of methods also serves the purpose of testing the robustness of the results. Some descriptions of the data set and methodology have naturally been repeated from chapter to chapter. Language and style might in some cases vary as the different chapters were written for the purpose of publication in various journals.

Chapter 2 focuses on income-related inequality in prescription medicine. Medicine is measured in terms of pharmacy retail prices and DDD. The horizontal inequity index is estimated by indirect standardization using a Two-Part model with need-based variables to predict the expected level of utilization. Data not weighted.

Chapter 3 is about income-related inequality in health care utilization. Six types of health care and aggregate health care utilization are measured in monetary terms. Horizontal inequity indices are estimated by indirect standardization using a Two-Part model with standardizing and non-standardizing variables to predict the expected level of utilization (where the non-standardizing variables have been set to their means). Data weighted by the reciprocals of the sampling probabilities.

In **Chapter 4** the horizontal inequity indices for health care utilization are standardized by the decomposition method. Linear partial effects for the decomposition are approximated by a Two-Part model. The overall income-related inequality in health care utilization is decomposed into contributions from standardizing and non-standardizing explanatory variables and the six different types of health care. Data weighted by the reciprocals of the sampling probabilities.

Chapter 5 focuses on income-related inequality in health. EQ-5D TTO-values are used to operationalize health. The overall income-related inequality in health is decomposed into contributions from the EQ-5D dimensions and from standardizing and non-standardizing variables. The partial effects for the decomposition are estimated by OLS regression. Data not weighted.

In **Chapter 6** the decomposition technique is applied on the SF-36 summary scores, PCS and MCS. The overall income-related inequality in health is decomposed into contributions from the SF-36 dimensions and from standardizing and non-standardizing variables. The partial effects for the decomposition are estimated by OLS regression. Data weighted by the reciprocals of the sampling probabilities. Data weighted by the reciprocals of the sampling probabilities.

A non-response analysis is carried out in **Chapter 7**. The bias for health care utilization estimates is quantified by comparing respondents with non-respondents and to classify the non-response bias into different types of non-response. The non-response bias from the Funen County Health Survey is compared to another Danish health survey. Data weighted by the reciprocals of the sampling probabilities.

** Appendix: Descriptive statistics**

Table A1. Mean health care costs for 2000 and 2001. The Funen County Health Survey

		Mean	CI 95% lower	CI 95% upper	Share of users	n	n$_{weighted}$
All	All	18102	16171	20033	0.98	2915	2915.0
Gender	Men	15701	13713	17689	0.97	1476	1491.8
	Women	20618	17263	23973	0.99	1439	1423.2
Age	16-24	12869	2857	22881	0.99	340	351.1
	25-44	13162	10813	15511	0.98	1152	1164.9
	45-66	19578	17062	22094	0.99	1111	1097.5
	67-80	37901	31379	44424	0.98	312	301.5
Income	0-99000	21716	15250	28182	0.98	625	640.1
	100000-199000	23155	19633	26677	0.98	890	864.2
	200000-299000	14475	12233	16717	0.98	929	929.0
	300000+	11229	9326	13131	0.98	471	481.7
Education	Low education	20307	17703	22910	0.98	1960	1895.3
	Medium education	17506	12259	22752	0.99	423	432.3
	High education	18772	12120	25424	0.97	161	184.6
	Other education	8057	6379	9736	0.98	371	402.8
Occupation	Unskilled	11438	8974	13902	0.99	311	278.9
	Skilled worker	10992	8684	13300	0.98	453	424.0
	White-collar	13736	11207	16264	0.98	839	895.7
	Selfemployed	15728	11325	20131	0.98	143	125.7
	Assisting spouse	7672	6313	9030	1.00	15	13.7
	Housewife	21271	10715	31827	1.00	43	41.3
	Student	6736	5284	8188	0.98	270	301.5
	Apprentice	9827	4734	14920	0.96	45	43.8
	Unemployed	50653	-6538	107844	1.00	63	62.0
	Retired	38391	32672	44110	0.98	559	549.1
	Other occupation	16570	11011	22128	0.99	174	179.1
Marital status	Married	19722	17564	21881	0.99	1654	1609.5
	Cohabitant	10902	8769	13035	0.98	431	426.7
	Alone	13661	7008	20314	0.97	527	561.1
	Divorced	29880	18134	41626	0.98	149	154.0
	Separated	24354	19219	29489	0.93	17	21.0
	Widowed	25825	18928	32721	0.97	132	137.5
	Other status	7802	6221	9383	1.00	5	5.2

Mean health care costs (hospital+GP+specialist+physiotherapy+dentistry+medicine) for 2000 and 2001 (both years included) measured in DKK, 2003 price level. Data weighted by the reciprocals of the sampling probabilities scaled to n (not taking item-non-response into account). 95% confidence intervals adjusted for the stratified sampling design. Share of users: Proportion of respondents with non-zero costs.

Table A2. Mean hospital costs for 2000 and 2001. The Funen County Health Survey

		Mean	CI 95% lower	CI 95% upper	Share of users	n	n$_{weighted}$
All	All	11502	9669	13335	0.43	2915	2915.0
Gender	Men	10150	8315	11984	0.41	1476	1491.8
	Women	12919	9698	16141	0.45	1439	1423.2
Age	16-24	9609	-294	19513	0.41	340	351.1
	25-44	8347	6101	10594	0.42	1152	1164.9
	45-66	11530	9268	13792	0.41	1111	1097.5
	67-80	25791	19648	31933	0.60	312	301.5
Income	0-99000	15282	8993	21571	0.45	625	640.1
	100000-199000	15227	11927	18528	0.48	890	864.2
	200000-299000	8611	6587	10634	0.42	929	929.0
	300000+	5372	3727	7017	0.33	471	481.7
Education	Low education	13106	10625	15586	0.45	1960	1895.3
	Medium education	11031	6034	16028	0.41	423	432.3
	High education	11729	5562	17896	0.41	161	184.6
	Other education	4358	2841	5875	0.40	371	402.8
Occupation	Unskilled	6237	4005	8469	0.38	311	278.9
	Skilled worker	6501	4390	8611	0.44	453	424.0
	White-collar	7662	5324	10000	0.38	839	895.7
	Selfemployed	9766	5514	14018	0.39	143	125.7
	Assisting spouse	2173	2031	2315	0.21	15	13.7
	Housewife	10385	2563	18207	0.46	43	41.3
	Student	3368	2124	4611	0.38	270	301.5
	Apprentice	6021	1406	10637	0.59	45	43.8
	Unemployed	41462	-15464	98388	0.55	63	62.0
	Retired	26794	21414	32174	0.55	559	549.1
	Other occupation	10726	5374	16078	0.42	174	179.1
Marital status	Married	12269	10285	14254	0.44	1654	1609.5
	Cohabitant	6163	4459	7867	0.43	431	426.7
	Alone	9638	3088	16187	0.38	527	561.1
	Divorced	21388	10109	32666	0.47	149	154.0
	Separated	17233	16705	17761	0.48	17	21.0
	Widowed	15116	8536	21696	0.49	132	137.5
	Other status	1626	1626	1626	0.45	5	5.2

Mean hospital costs (DRG-charges) for 2000 and 2001 (both years included) measured in DKK, 2003 price level. Data weighted by the reciprocals of the sampling probabilities scaled to n (not taking item-non-response into account). 95% confidence intervals adjusted for the stratified sampling design. Share of users: Proportion of respondents with non-zero costs.

Table A3. Mean GP costs for 2000 and 2001. The Funen County Health Survey

		Mean	CI 95% lower	CI 95% upper	Share of users	n	n_weighted
All	All	1639	1568	1710	0.93	2915	2915.0
Gender	Men	1215	1133	1297	0.89	1476	1491.8
	Women	2083	1970	2196	0.97	1439	1423.2
Age	16-24	1342	1175	1508	0.94	340	351.1
	25-44	1452	1357	1548	0.93	1152	1164.9
	45-66	1646	1529	1763	0.92	1111	1097.5
	67-80	2679	2352	3005	0.95	312	301.5
Income	0-99000	1924	1738	2109	0.94	625	640.1
	100000-199000	1941	1811	2072	0.95	890	864.2
	200000-299000	1459	1343	1576	0.92	929	929.0
	300000+	1064	944	1184	0.89	471	481.7
Education	Low education	1755	1663	1847	0.93	1960	1895.3
	Medium education	1422	1257	1587	0.93	423	432.3
	High education	1393	1118	1667	0.89	161	184.6
	Other education	1439	1264	1614	0.93	371	402.8
Occupation	Unskilled	1558	1351	1764	0.94	311	278.9
	Skilled worker	1261	1133	1388	0.91	453	424.0
	White-collar	1443	1328	1558	0.92	839	895.7
	Selfemployed	1142	946	1338	0.89	143	125.7
	Assisting spouse	1282	821	1743	0.88	15	13.7
	Housewife	2398	1762	3035	0.97	43	41.3
	Student	1460	1249	1670	0.94	270	301.5
	Apprentice	1148	859	1436	0.92	45	43.8
	Unemployed	2236	1717	2755	0.97	63	62.0
	Retired	2474	2247	2700	0.95	559	549.1
	Other occupation	1496	1256	1736	0.93	174	179.1
Marital status	Married	1661	1565	1757	0.94	1654	1609.5
	Cohabitant	1465	1304	1626	0.92	431	426.7
	Alone	1354	1215	1493	0.92	527	561.1
	Divorced	2214	1794	2634	0.96	149	154.0
	Separated	2233	1356	3111	0.93	17	21.0
	Widowed	2352	1945	2759	0.93	132	137.5
	Other status	1560	582	2538	1.00	5	5.2

Mean GP costs (fees + average rate of capitation) for 2000 and 2001 (both years included) measured in DKK, 2003 price level. Data weighted by the reciprocals of the sampling probabilities scaled to n (not taking item-non-response into account). 95% confidence intervals adjusted for the stratified sampling design. Share of users: Proportion of respondents with non-zero costs.

Table A4. Mean specialist costs for 2000 and 2001. The Funen County Health Survey

		Mean	CI 95% lower	CI 95% upper	Share of users	n	n_weighted
All	All	578	506	650	0.36	2915	2915.0
Gender	Men	473	366	580	0.31	1476	1491.8
	Women	688	592	784	0.42	1439	1423.2
Age	16-24	367	253	482	0.29	340	351.1
	25-44	456	341	571	0.31	1152	1164.9
	45-66	672	541	802	0.40	1111	1097.5
	67-80	956	753	1158	0.54	312	301.5
Income	0-99000	602	434	770	0.37	625	640.1
	100000-199000	702	576	829	0.43	890	864.2
	200000-299000	434	347	521	0.33	929	929.0
	300000+	600	357	844	0.31	471	481.7
Education	Low education	600	514	686	0.38	1960	1895.3
	Medium education	631	367	896	0.36	423	432.3
	High education	701	388	1013	0.39	161	184.6
	Other education	360	274	446	0.30	371	402.8
Occupation	Unskilled	479	359	599	0.36	311	278.9
	Skilled worker	262	204	320	0.27	453	424.0
	White-collar	629	462	796	0.33	839	895.7
	Selfemployed	507	334	679	0.38	143	125.7
	Assisting spouse	287	-150	724	0.36	15	13.7
	Housewife	776	401	1151	0.55	43	41.3
	Student	336	238	434	0.29	270	301.5
	Apprentice	402	201	604	0.36	45	43.8
	Unemployed	574	298	850	0.43	63	62.0
	Retired	913	696	1129	0.50	559	549.1
	Other occupation	676	364	989	0.40	174	179.1
Marital status	Married	675	567	782	0.40	1654	1609.5
	Cohabitant	411	217	605	0.29	431	426.7
	Alone	408	279	536	0.28	527	561.1
	Divorced	589	408	771	0.41	149	154.0
	Separated	643	-31	1317	0.43	17	21.0
	Widowed	658	472	844	0.48	132	137.5
	Other status	0	0	0	0.00	5	5.2

Mean specialist costs (fees) for 2000 and 2001 (both years included) measured in DKK, 2003 price level. Data weighted by the reciprocals of the sampling probabilities scaled to n (not taking item-non-response into account). 95% confidence intervals adjusted for the stratified sampling design. Share of users: Proportion of respondents with non-zero costs.

Table A5. Mean physiotherapist costs for 2000 and 2001. The Funen County Health Survey

		Mean	CI 95% lower	CI 95% upper	Share of users	n	n_weighted
All	All	395	307	483	0.11	2915	2915.0
Gender	Men	330	215	444	0.09	1476	1491.8
	Women	464	329	598	0.13	1439	1423.2
Age	16-24	191	-3	385	0.05	340	351.1
	25-44	265	176	353	0.10	1152	1164.9
	45-66	451	291	612	0.12	1111	1097.5
	67-80	931	481	1381	0.18	312	301.5
Income	0-99000	389	208	570	0.11	625	640.1
	100000-199000	450	292	609	0.12	890	864.2
	200000-299000	428	238	617	0.10	929	929.0
	300000+	241	133	348	0.10	471	481.7
Education	Low education	401	294	507	0.11	1960	1895.3
	Medium education	574	266	881	0.12	423	432.3
	High education	425	101	748	0.11	161	184.6
	Other education	162	37	288	0.07	371	402.8
Occupation	Unskilled	124	37	210	0.06	311	278.9
	Skilled worker	183	92	275	0.10	453	424.0
	White-collar	254	180	327	0.11	839	895.7
	Selfemployed	495	-136	1126	0.10	143	125.7
	Assisting spouse	1145	641	1648	0.20	15	13.7
	Housewife	429	-47	905	0.16	43	41.3
	Student	162	-1	325	0.05	270	301.5
	Apprentice	841	-502	2184	0.21	45	43.8
	Unemployed	930	30	1831	0.11	63	62.0
	Retired	945	582	1308	0.17	559	549.1
	Other occupation	304	58	549	0.09	174	179.1
Marital status	Married	439	322	556	0.13	1654	1609.5
	Cohabitant	305	106	503	0.08	431	426.7
	Alone	270	104	435	0.08	527	561.1
	Divorced	470	-58	998	0.07	149	154.0
	Separated	805	-744	2354	0.09	17	21.0
	Widowed	539	-66	1145	0.11	132	137.5
	Other status	0	0	0	0.00	5	5.2

Mean physiotherapist costs (fees + copayment) for 2000 and 2001 (both years included) measured in DKK, 2003 price level. Data weighted by the reciprocals of the sampling probabilities scaled to n (not taking item-non-response into account). 95% confidence intervals adjusted for the stratified sampling design. Share of users: Proportion of respondents with non-zero costs.

Table A6. Mean dentist costs for 2000 and 2001. The Funen County Health Survey

		Mean	CI 95% lower	CI 95% upper	Share of users	n	n$_{weighted}$
All	All	1680	1618	1742	0.79	2915	2915.0
Gender	Men	1643	1554	1732	0.77	1476	1491.8
	Women	1719	1633	1805	0.82	1439	1423.2
Age	16-24	936	807	1066	0.69	340	351.1
	25-44	1600	1504	1696	0.82	1152	1164.9
	45-66	2093	1992	2194	0.85	1111	1097.5
	67-80	1355	1157	1552	0.60	312	301.5
Income	0-99000	1109	1001	1217	0.66	625	640.1
	100000-199000	1759	1645	1873	0.81	890	864.2
	200000-299000	1791	1684	1897	0.85	929	929.0
	300000+	2086	1918	2254	0.85	471	481.7
Education	Low education	1702	1626	1778	0.78	1960	1895.3
	Medium education	2074	1904	2243	0.90	423	432.3
	High education	1783	1529	2036	0.82	161	184.6
	Other education	1108	970	1246	0.72	371	402.8
Occupation	Unskilled	1658	1439	1876	0.77	311	278.9
	Skilled worker	1602	1462	1742	0.82	453	424.0
	White-collar	1946	1833	2059	0.89	839	895.7
	Selfemployed	2103	1790	2415	0.85	143	125.7
	Assisting spouse	1766	1546	1985	0.93	15	13.7
	Housewife	2288	1725	2852	0.95	43	41.3
	Student	943	816	1069	0.69	270	301.5
	Apprentice	1012	660	1364	0.73	45	43.8
	Unemployed	1906	1439	2373	0.77	63	62.0
	Retired	1593	1442	1743	0.67	559	549.1
	Other occupation	1725	1483	1967	0.80	174	179.1
Marital status	Married	1902	1818	1985	0.84	1654	1609.5
	Cohabitant	1513	1360	1665	0.81	431	426.7
	Alone	1128	1010	1246	0.70	527	561.1
	Divorced	1912	1626	2198	0.76	149	154.0
	Separated	1408	755	2061	0.76	17	21.0
	Widowed	1672	1338	2007	0.64	132	137.5
	Other status	889	-63	1840	0.55	5	5.2

Mean dentist costs (fees + approximated co-payment) for 2000 and 2001 (both years included) measured in DKK, 2003 price level. Data weighted by the reciprocals of the sampling probabilities scaled to n (not taking item-non-response into account). 95% confidence intervals adjusted for the stratified sampling design. Share of users: Proportion of respondents with non-zero costs.

Table A7. Mean prescription medicine costs for 2000 and 2001. The Funen County Health Survey

			CI 95%		Share		
		Mean	lower	upper	of users	n	n_weighted
All	All	2307	2093	2522	0.75	2915	2915.0
Gender	Men	1890	1629	2151	0.67	1476	1491.8
	Women	2745	2401	3089	0.82	1439	1423.2
Age	16-24	424	295	552	0.66	340	351.1
	25-44	1042	839	1245	0.71	1152	1164.9
	45-66	3186	2779	3593	0.77	1111	1097.5
	67-80	6191	5149	7232	0.88	312	301.5
Income	0-99000	2410	1969	2852	0.74	625	640.1
	100000-199000	3075	2599	3550	0.81	890	864.2
	200000-299000	1752	1440	2065	0.73	929	929.0
	300000+	1865	1369	2362	0.68	471	481.7
Education	Low education	2743	2447	3040	0.77	1960	1895.3
	Medium education	1774	1413	2135	0.72	423	432.3
	High education	2742	1650	3833	0.73	161	184.6
	Other education	630	476	784	0.67	371	402.8
Occupation	Unskilled	1383	992	1774	0.77	311	278.9
	Skilled worker	1183	843	1524	0.66	453	424.0
	White-collar	1803	1429	2176	0.73	839	895.7
	Selfemployed	1715	1046	2385	0.73	143	125.7
	Assisting spouse	1019	-81	2119	0.75	15	13.7
	Housewife	4995	2006	7983	0.92	43	41.3
	Student	467	334	601	0.67	270	301.5
	Apprentice	402	105	700	0.61	45	43.8
	Unemployed	3544	1404	5685	0.83	63	62.0
	Retired	5674	4942	6406	0.87	559	549.1
	Other occupation	1643	1144	2142	0.71	174	179.1
Marital status	Married	2777	2469	3085	0.78	1654	1609.5
	Cohabitant	1045	574	1516	0.69	431	426.7
	Alone	865	672	1057	0.67	527	561.1
	Divorced	3306	2219	4393	0.79	149	154.0
	Separated	2032	-248	4313	0.70	17	21.0
	Widowed	5488	3941	7035	0.84	132	137.5
	Other status	3728	3380	4076	0.61	5	5.2

Mean prescription medicine costs (retail sales prices) for 2000 and 2001 (both years included) measured in DKK, 2003 price level. Data weighted by the reciprocals of the sampling probabilities scaled to n (not taking item-non-response into account). 95% confidence intervals adjusted for the stratified sampling design. Share of users: Proportion of respondents with non-zero costs.

Table A8. Mean EQ-5D TTO value. The Funen County Health Survey

		Mean	CI 95% lower	CI 95% upper	Share with problems	n	n_weighted
All	All	0.90	0.89	0.90	0.40	2915	2915.0
Gender	Men	0.91	0.90	0.92	0.36	1476	1491.8
	Women	0.88	0.87	0.89	0.46	1439	1423.2
Age	16-24	0.94	0.92	0.95	0.27	340	351.1
	25-44	0.91	0.90	0.92	0.38	1152	1164.9
	45-66	0.88	0.87	0.89	0.43	1111	1097.5
	67-80	0.84	0.82	0.87	0.55	312	301.5
Income	0-99000	0.88	0.87	0.90	0.43	625	640.1
	100000-199000	0.87	0.85	0.88	0.49	890	864.2
	200000-299000	0.91	0.90	0.92	0.36	929	929.0
	300000+	0.94	0.93	0.95	0.29	471	481.7
Education	Low education	0.88	0.87	0.89	0.44	1960	1895.3
	Medium education	0.91	0.90	0.93	0.38	423	432.3
	High education	0.93	0.92	0.95	0.31	161	184.6
	Other education	0.93	0.91	0.94	0.32	371	402.8
Occupation	Unskilled	0.91	0.89	0.92	0.40	311	278.9
	Skilled worker	0.91	0.89	0.92	0.39	453	424.0
	White-collar	0.92	0.91	0.93	0.35	839	895.7
	Selfemployed	0.93	0.91	0.95	0.31	143	125.7
	Assisting spouse	0.90	0.83	0.98	0.46	15	13.7
	Housewife	0.83	0.78	0.89	0.58	43	41.3
	Student	0.94	0.92	0.95	0.29	270	301.5
	Apprentice	0.91	0.88	0.95	0.42	45	43.8
	Unemployed	0.83	0.77	0.90	0.51	63	62.0
	Retired	0.83	0.81	0.85	0.57	559	549.1
	Other occupation	0.88	0.85	0.90	0.43	174	179.1
Marital status	Married	0.89	0.88	0.90	0.42	1654	1609.5
	Cohabitant	0.92	0.91	0.94	0.32	431	426.7
	Alone	0.92	0.91	0.93	0.35	527	561.1
	Divorced	0.85	0.81	0.88	0.49	149	154.0
	Separated	0.80	0.70	0.91	0.57	17	21.0
	Widowed	0.84	0.80	0.88	0.53	132	137.5
	Other status	0.85	0.00	1.70	0.73	5	5.2

Mean EQ-5D scores evaluated with TTO-values. Scale: 1 perfect health, 0 death, negative values possible. Data weighted by the reciprocals of the sampling probabilities scaled to n (not taking item non-response into account). 95% confidence intervals adjusted for the stratified sampling design. Share with problems: Proportion of respondents with problems reported in at least one EQ-5D dimension.

Table A9. Mean PCS and MCS scores. The Funen County Health Survey

		Mean score			
		PCS	MCS	n	n_weighted
All	All	51.83	56.10	2759	2768.0
Gender	Men	52.11	57.17	1401	1415.3
	Women	51.53	54.97	1358	1352.7
Age	16-24	54.10	55.89	330	340.1
	25-44	53.24	55.50	1093	1108.9
	45-66	50.89	56.46	1046	1036.8
	67-80	46.98	57.36	290	282.2
Income	0-99000	50.22	55.83	592	608.1
	100000-199000	51.00	55.15	839	817.5
	200000-299000	52.69	56.50	885	889.1
	300000+	53.76	57.36	443	453.2
Education	Low education	51.08	56.10	1851	1796.8
	Medium education	52.84	56.54	402	411.8
	High education	53.39	56.41	151	172.7
	Other education	53.51	55.45	355	386.7
Occupation	Unskilled	52.53	56.38	295	264.8
	Skilled worker	52.47	56.77	435	408.8
	White-collar	53.59	56.01	793	849.0
	Selfemployed	53.03	57.57	132	117.0
	Assisting spouse	50.59	56.07	15	13.7
	Housewife	48.86	52.90	39	37.4
	Student	54.12	55.24	261	291.3
	Apprentice	51.71	58.03	43	41.4
	Unemployed	49.49	53.44	59	59.1
	Retired	47.00	56.36	528	521.7
	Other occupation	51.99	55.26	159	163.8
Marital status	Married	51.42	56.70	1554	1517.1
	Cohabitant	53.39	56.21	417	415.3
	Alone	53.31	55.44	507	538.8
	Divorced	49.40	53.61	140	145.3
	Separated	51.62	51.57	14	17.3
	Widowed	48.22	54.65	122	129.0
	Other status	50.23	59.52	5	5.2

PCS: Physical Component Score, MCS: Mental Component Score. Scale: Standardized to the American norm of a mean of 50 and a standard deviation of 10. Data weighted by the reciprocals of the sampling probabilities (not taking item non-response into account. The lower number of respondents (compared to the other tables) is caused by a higher number of item non-respondents for the PCS and MCS calculations.

Table A10. Proportion of respondents with life-style characteristics. The Funen County Health Survey

		Daily smoker	High alcohol	Cooked vegetables	Raw vegetables	Daily fruit	No exercises	n	$n_{weighted}$
All	All	0.36	0.10	0.29	0.29	0.59	0.10	2915	2915.0
Gender	Men	0.37	0.14	0.25	0.21	0.47	0.11	1476	1491.8
	Women	0.34	0.07	0.35	0.37	0.72	0.10	1439	1423.2
Age	16-24	0.27	0.19	0.17	0.28	0.47	0.07	340	351.1
	25-44	0.37	0.08	0.27	0.32	0.54	0.10	1152	1164.9
	45-66	0.38	0.11	0.32	0.28	0.66	0.11	1111	1097.5
	67-80	0.31	0.09	0.43	0.20	0.74	0.15	312	301.5
Income	0-99000	0.33	0.11	0.26	0.24	0.58	0.12	625	640.1
	100000-199000	0.40	0.09	0.32	0.28	0.65	0.11	890	864.2
	200000-299000	0.37	0.10	0.28	0.31	0.57	0.10	929	929.0
	300000+	0.27	0.13	0.31	0.31	0.58	0.09	471	481.7
Education	Low education	0.41	0.10	0.29	0.24	0.59	0.12	1960	1895.3
	Medium education	0.28	0.10	0.37	0.44	0.68	0.07	423	432.3
	High education	0.25	0.15	0.34	0.42	0.63	0.08	161	184.6
	Other education	0.24	0.12	0.21	0.29	0.51	0.05	371	402.8
Occupation	Unskilled	0.50	0.08	0.21	0.22	0.48	0.09	311	278.9
	Skilled worker	0.40	0.09	0.21	0.21	0.49	0.10	453	424.0
	White-collar	0.30	0.11	0.34	0.39	0.65	0.08	839	895.7
	Selfemployed	0.35	0.13	0.38	0.24	0.52	0.16	143	125.7
	Assisting spouse	0.15	0.10	0.27	0.14	0.82	0.12	15	13.7
	Housewife	0.38	0.11	0.38	0.29	0.79	0.18	43	41.3
	Student	0.22	0.12	0.20	0.33	0.50	0.04	270	301.5
	Apprentice	0.36	0.31	0.07	0.09	0.35	0.14	45	43.8
	Unemployed	0.62	0.14	0.28	0.23	0.56	0.14	63	62.0
	Retired	0.38	0.08	0.39	0.20	0.71	0.16	559	549.1
	Other occupation	0.39	0.07	0.27	0.38	0.65	0.11	174	179.1
Marital status	Married	0.34	0.08	0.34	0.30	0.65	0.10	1654	1609.5
	Cohabitant	0.38	0.10	0.25	0.27	0.51	0.09	431	426.7
	Alone	0.34	0.17	0.19	0.25	0.47	0.09	527	561.1
	Divorced	0.49	0.09	0.25	0.29	0.58	0.18	149	154.0
	Separated	0.53	0.18	0.28	0.31	0.51	0.15	17	21.0
	Widowed	0.37	0.10	0.39	0.28	0.75	0.11	132	137.5
	Other status	0.37	0.10	0.22	0.24	0.73	0.10	5	5.2

Proportion of respondents reporting yes to certain life-style characteristics. Data weighted by the reciprocals of the sampling probabilities scaled to n (not taking item non-response into account).

References

1. Wagstaff A, van Doorslaer E. Equity in Health Care Finance and Delivery. *Handbook of health economics. Volume 1B* 2000;1803-62.

2. Williams A. Intergenerational equity: an exploration of the 'fair innings' argument. *Health Econ* 1997;**6**:117-32.

3. Olsen JA. Theories of justice and their implications for priority setting in health care. *J Health Econ* 1997;**16**:625-39.

4. Nord E, Pinto JL, Richardson J, Menzel P, Ubel P. Incorporating societal concerns for fairness in numerical valuations of health programmes. *Health Econ* 1999;**8**:25-39.

5. Williams AH, Cookson RA. Equity-efficiency trade-offs in health technology assessment. *Int J Technol Assess Health Care* 2006;**22**:1-9.

6. Hurley J. An Overview of the Normative Economics of the Health Sector. *Handbook of health economics. Volume 1A* 2000;55-118.

7. Tobin J. Limiting Domain of Inequality. *J Law & Econ* 1970;**13**:263-77.

8. Elster J. *Local Justice: How Institutions Allocate Scarce Goods and Necessary Burdens*. Russell Sage Foundation, 1992.

9. Musgrave RA. *The Theory of Public Finance: A study in Public Economy*. New York, Toronto, London: McGraw-Hill, 1959.

10. Daniels N. *Just Health Care*. Cambridge: Cambridge University Press, 1985.

11. Culyer AJ, Wagstaff A. Equity and Equality in Health and Health Care. *J Health Econ* 1993;**12**:431-57.

12. Wagstaff A, van Doorslaer E. Equity in the Finance and Delivery of Health Care: Concepts and Definitions. In: van Doorslaer E, Wagstaff A, Rutten F, editors. *Equity in the Finance and Delivery of Health Care*. Oxford University Press, 1993.

13. Wagstaff A. QALYs and the equity-efficiency trade-off. *J Health Econ* 1991;**10**:21-41.

14. Sen A. *Inequality Reexamined*. Oxford University Press, 1992.

15. Sen A. Why health equity? *Health Econ* 2002;**11**:659-66.

16. Culyer AJ, van Doorslaer E, Wagstaff A. Utilisation as a measure of equity by Mooney, Hall, Donaldson and Gerard. *J Health Econ* 1992;**11**:93-98.

17. Culyer AJ, van Doorslaer E, Wagstaff A. Access, Utilisation and Equity: A Further Comment. *J Health Econ* 1992;**11**:207-10.

18. Culyer AJ, van Doorslaer E, Wagstaff A. Utilisation as a Measure of Equity: Comment. *J Health Econ* 1992;**11**:93-98.

19. Mooney G, Hall J, Donaldson C, Gerard K. Utilisation as a measure of equity: weighing heat? *J Health Econ* 1991;**10**:475-80.

20. Mooney G, Hall J, Donaldson C, Gerard K. Reweighing heat: response to Culyer, van Doorslaer and Wagstaff. *J Health Econ* 1992;**11**:199-205.

21. Le Grand J. Equity. In: Health, and Health Care. *Social Justice Research* 1987;**1**:257-74.

22. Mooney G. Equity. *Key Issues in Health Economics*. New York: Wheatsheaf, 1994:65-86.

23. Williams A. Economics, Society and health Care Ethics. In: Gillon R, editor. *Principles of Health Care Ethics*. John Wiley & sons, 1994.

24. Culyer AJ. Equity - some theory and its policy implications. *J Med Ethics* 2001;**27**:275-83.

25. Culyer AJ. Health, Health Expenditures and Equity. In: van Doorslaer E, Wagstaff A, Rutten F, editors. *Equity in the Finance and Delivery of Health Care: An International Perspective*. Oxford University Press, 1993.

26. Hurley J. Ethics, economics, and public financing of health care. *J Med Ethics* 2001;**27**:234-39.

27. Donabedian A. Evaluating the Quality of Medical Care. *The Milbank Memorial Fund Quarterly* 1966;**44**:166-203.

28. Culyer AJ. The Normative Economics of Health Care Finance and Provision. *Oxford Review of Economic Policy* 1989;**5**:34-55.

29. Beauchamp TL. The 'Four Principles' Approach. In: Gillon R, editor. *Principles of Health Care Ethics*. John Wiley & sons, 1994.

30. Gillon R. *Philosophical Medical Ethics*. John Wiley & sons, 1985.

31. Gillon R. Preface: Medical Ethics and the Four Principles. In: Gillon R, editor. *Principles of Health Care Ethics.* John Wiley & sons, 1994.

32. Williams A, Cookson R. Equity in Health. *Handbook of health economics. Volume 1B* 2000;1863-910.

33. Bentham J. *An Introduction to the Principles of Morals and Legislation.* Blackwell Publishing, 1789.

34. Mill JS. *Utililtarianism.* Blackwell Publishing, 1861.

35. Sen A, Willams B. Introduction: Utilitarianism and beyond. In: Sen A, Williams B, editors. *Utilitarianism and Beyond.* Paris: Cambridge Univeristy Press, 1982.

36. Hammond PJ. Utilitarianism, uncertainty and information. In: Sen A, Williams B, editors. *Utilitarianism and Beyond.* Paris: Cambridge Univeristy Press, 1982.

37. Harsanyi JC. Morality and the theory of rational behaviour. In: Sen A, Williams B, editors. *Utilitarianism and Beyond.* Paris: Cambridge Univeristy Press, 1982.

38. Hare RM. Ethical theory and utilitarianism. In: Sen A, Williams B, editors. *Utilitarianism and Beyond.* Paris: Cambridge Univeristy Press, 1982.

39. Harsanyi JC. Cardinal utility in welfare economics and in the theory of risk-taking. *J Pol Econ* 1953;**61**:434-35.

40. Harsanyi JC. Can the Maximin Principle Serve as a Basis for Morality? A Critique of John Rawls's Theory. *American Pol Science Rev* 1975;**69**:594-606.

41. Nozick R. *Anarchy, State, and Utopia.* Blackwell Publishing, 1974.

42. Hausman DM, Mcpherson MS. Taking Ethics Seriously - Economics and Contemporary Moral-Philosophy. *J Econ Literature* 1993;**31**:671-731.

43. Rawls J. *A Theory of Justice.* The Belknap Press of Harvard University Press, 1971.

44. Rawls J. Social unity and primary goods. In: Sen A, Williams B, editors. *Utilitarianism and Beyond.* Paris: Cambridge Univeristy Press, 1982.

45. Rawls J. *Political Liberalism.* Expanded edition ed. New York: Columbia University Press, 1993.

46. Arrow KJ. Some Ordinalist-Utilitarian Notes on Rawls's Theory of Justice. *J Philosophy* 1973;**70**:245-63.

47. Andersen RM. Revisiting the Behavioral-Model and Access to Medical-Care - Does It Matter? *J Health Soc Behavior* 1995;1-10.

48. Le Grand J. *The Strategy of Equality.* London: Unwin Hyman, 1982.

49. Olsen EO, Rogers DL. The welfare economics of equal access. *J Public Econ* 1991;**45**:91-105.

50. McGuire A, Henderson J, Mooney G. *The Economics of Health care: An Introductory Text.* Routledge & Kegan Paul, 1988.

51. Tsuchiya A, Williams A. A "fair innings" between the sexes: are men being treated inequitably? *Soc Sci Med* 2005;**60**:277-86.

52. Vallgarda S. When are health inequalities a political problem? *Eur J Public Health* 2006;**16**:615-16.

53. Harris J. *Value of Life: An Introduction to Medical Ethics*. Taylor and Francis e-Library, 2001, 1985.

54. Stolk EA, van DG, Brouwer WB, Busschbach JJ. Reconciliation of economic concerns and health policy: illustration of an equity adjustment procedure using proportional shortfall. *Pharmacoeconomics* 2004;**22**:1097-107.

55. Stolk EA, Pickee SJ, Ament AH, Busschbach JJ. Equity in health care prioritisation: an empirical inquiry into social value. *Health Policy* 2005;**74**:343-55.

56. Dolan PA, Olsen JA. Equity in health: the importance of different health streams. *J Health Econ* 2001;**20**:823-34.

57. Anand P. Capabilities and Health. *J Med Ethics* 2005;**31**:299-303.

58. Williams A. Comment on Amartya Sen's 'Why Health Equity'. *Health Econ* 2003;**12**:65-66.

59. Calabresi G, Bobbit P. *Tragic Choices*. Norton, 1978.

60. Grossman M. On the Concept of Health Capital and the Demand for Health. *J Political Econ* 1972;**80**:223-55.

61. Grossman M. *The Demand for Health: A Theoretical and Empirical Investigation*. 119. 1972. New York, National Bureau of Economic Research. Occational paper.

62. Grossman M. The Human Capital Model. *Handbook of health economics. Volume 1A* 2000;347-408.

63. Muurinen JM, Le Grand J. The economic analysis of inequalities in health. *Soc Sci Med* 1985;**20**:1029-35.

64. Chang FR. Uncertainty and investment in Health. *J Health Econ* 1996;**15**:369-76.

65. Cropper ML. Health, Investment in Health, and Occupational Choice. *J Political Econ* 1977;**85**:1273-94.

66. Dardanoni V, Wagstaff A. Uncertainty, inequalities in health and the demand for health. *J Health Econ* 1987;**6**:283-90.

67. Dardanoni V, Wagstaff A. Uncertainty and the demand for medical care. *J Health Econ* 1990;**9**:23-38.

68. Mooney G, Ryan M. Agency in health care: getting beyond first principles. *J Health Econ* 1993;**12**:125-35.

69. Gafni A, Charles C, Whelan T. The physician-patient encounter: the physician as a perfect agent for the patient versus the informed treatment decision-making model. *Soc Sci Med* 1998;**47**:347-54.

70. Veatch RM. Doctor does not know best: why in the new century physicians must stop trying to benefit patients. *J Med Philos* 2000;**25**:701-21.

71. Reinhardt UE. The theory of physician induced demand. Reflections after a decade. *J Health Econ* 1985;**4**:187-93.

72. Evans RG. Supplier induced demand: some evidence and some implications. In: Perlman M, editor. *The Economics of Health and Medical Care*. New York: Macmillan, 1974.

73. Stano M. A Clarification of Theories and Evidence on Supplier-Induced Demand for Physicians' Services. *J Human Res* 1987;**22**:611-20.

74. Labelle R, Stoddart GL, Rice T. A re-examination of the meaning and importance of supplier-induced demand. *J Health Econ* 1994;**13**:347-68.

75. Hay J, Leahy MJ. Physician induced demand. An empirical analysis of the consumer informaton gap. *J Health Econ* 1982;**1**:231-44.

76. Rice T. *The Economics of Health Reconsidered*. Chicago: AHSR, 1998.

77. Jessor R. Risk behavior in adolescence: a psychosocial framework for understanding and action. *J Adolesc Health* 1991;**12**:597-605.

78. Lynam MJ. Health as a socially mediated process: theoretical and practice imperatives emerging from research on health inequalities. *ANS Adv Nurs Sci* 2005;**28**:25-37.

79. Rose G. *The Strategy of Preventive Medicine*. Oxford University Press, 1992.

80. Sampson RJ. The neighborhood context of well-being. *Perspect Biol Med* 2003;**46**:S53-S64.

81. Wold B, Øygard L, Eder A, Smith C. Social reproduction of physical activity. *Eur J Health Econ* 1994;**4**:163-68.

82. Aday LA. Economic and Noneconomic Barriers to the Use of Needed Medical Services. *Med Care* 1975;**13**:447-56.

83. Aday LA, Andersen RM. Equity of Access to Medical-Care - A Conceptual and Empirical Overview. *Med Care* 1981;**19**:4-27.

84. Andersen RM, McCutcheon A, Aday LA, Chiu GY, Bell R. Exploring Dimensions of Access to Medical-Care. *Health Serv Res* 1983;49-74.

85. Zere E, McIntyre D. Inequities in under-five child malnutrition in South Africa. *Int J Equity Health* 2003;**2**.

86. Van der Heyden JH, Demarest S, Tafforeau J, Van Oyen H. Socio-economic differences in the utilisation of health services in Belgium. *Health Policy* 2003;**65**:153-65.

87. van der Meer JB, van den Bos J, Mackenbach JP. Socioeconomic differences in the utilization of health services in a Dutch population: the contribution of health status. *Health Policy* 1996;**37**:1-18.

88. van Doorslaer E, Wagstaff A, van der Burg H, Christiansen T, De Graeve D, Duchesne I, Gerdtham UG, Gerfin M, Geurts J, Gross L, Häkkinen U, John J, Klavus J, Leu RE, Nolan B, O'Donnell O, Propper C, Puffer F, Schellhorn M, Sundberg G, Winkelhake O. Equity in the delivery of health care in Europe and the US. *J Health Econ* 2000;**19**:553-83.

89. van Doorslaer E, Masseria C and the OECD Health Equity Research Group Members. Income-Related Inequality in the Use of Medical Care in 21 OECD Countries. 14. 2004. Paris, OECD. OECD Health working papers.

90. Morris S, Sutton M, Gravelle H. Inequity and inequality in the use of health care in England: an empirical investigation. *Soc Sci Med* 2005;**60**:1251-66.

91. Gravelle H. Measuring income related inequality in health: standardisation and the partial concentration index. *Health Econ* 2003;**12**:803-19.

92. van Doorslaer E, Koolman X. Explaining the differences in income-related health inequalities across European countries. *Health Econ* 2004;**13**:609-28.

93. Kokko H, Mackenzie A, Reynolds JD, Lindstrom J, Sutherland WJ. Measures of Inequality Are Not Equal. *Am Nat* 1999;**154**:358-82.

94. Wagstaff A, van Doorslaer E. Overall versus socioeconomic health inequality: a measurement framework and two empirical illustrations. *Health Econ* 2004;**13**:297-301.

95. Williams RFG, Doessel DP. Measuring Inequality: tools and an illustration. *Int J Equity Health* 2006;**5**.

96. Allison PD. Measures of Inequality. *American Sociological Rev* 1978;**43**:865-80.

97. Mackenbach JP, Kunst AE. Measuring the magnitude of socio-economic inequalities in health: an overview of available measures illustrated with two examples from Europe. *Soc Sci Med* 1997;**44**:757-71.

98. Schneider MC, Castillo-Salgado C, Bacallao J, Loyola E, Mujica OJ, Vidaurre M, Roca A. Methods for measuring health inequalities (Part I). *Epidemiol Bull* 2004;**25**.

99. Sen A. *On Economic Inequality*. Enlarged edition with a substantial annexe 'On Economic Inequality after a Quarter Century' ed. Clarendon Press, 1997.

100. Wagstaff A, Paci P, van Doorslaer E. On the measurement of inequalities in health. *Soc Sci Med* 1991;**33**:545-57.

101. Asada Y. A framework for measuring health inequity. *J Epidemiol Community Health* 2005;**59**:700-705.

102. Chen AY, Escarce JJ. Quantifying income-related inequality in healthcare delivery in the United States. *Med Care* 2004;**42**:38-47.

103. Hosseinpoor AR, van Doorslaer E, Speybroeck N, Naghavi M, Mohammad K, Majdzadeh R, Delavar B, Jamshidi H, Vega J. Decomposing socioeconomic inequality in infant mortality in Iran. *Int J Epidemiol* 2006;**35**:1211-19.

104. Mangalore R, Knapp M, Jenkins R. Income-related inequality in mental health in Britain: the concentration index approach. *Psychol Med* 2007;1-9.

105. Nguyen L, Häkkinen U. Income-Related Inequality in the Use of Dental Services in Finland. *Appl Health Econ Health Policy* 2004;**3**:251-62.

106. van Doorslaer E, Wagstaff A, Calonge S, Christiansen T, Gerfin M, Gottschalk P, Janssen R, Lauchaud C, Leu RE, Nolan B, O'Donnel O, Paci P, Pereira J, Pinto CG, Propper C, Reñé J, Rochaix L, Rodríguez M, Rutten F, Upward R, Wolfe B. Equity in the delivery of health care: some international comparisons. *J Health Econ* 1992;**11**:389-411.

107. van Doorslaer E, Wagstaff A, Bleichrodt H, Calonge S, Gerdtham UG, Gerfin, M, Geurts J, Gross L, Häkkinen U, Leu RE, O'Donnell O, Propper C, Puffer F, Rodríguez M, Sundberg G, Winkelhake O. Income-related inequalities in health: some international comparisons. *J Health Econ* 1997;**16**:93-112.

108. Zhang Q, Wang Y. Socioeconomic inequlity of obesity in the United States: do gender, age, and ethnicity matter? *Soc Sci Med* 2004;**58**:1171-80.

109. Humphries KH, van Doorslaer E. Income-related health inequality in Canada. *Soc Sci Med* 2000;**50**:663-71.

110. Koolman X, van Doorslaer E. On the interpretation of a concentration index of inequality. *Health Econ* 2004;**13**:649-56.

111. Kakwani N, Wagstaff A, van Doorslaer E. Socioeconomic Inequalities in Health: Measurement, Computation, and Statistical Inference. *J Econometrics* 1997;**77**:87-103.

112. Lerman RI, Yitzhaki S. Improving the Accuracy of Estimates of Gini-Coefficients. *J Econometrics* 1989;**42**:43-47.

113. The World Bank. Technical Note #7: The Concentration Index. 2003. *Quantitative Techniques for Health Equity Analysis*.

114. Kakwani NC, Podder N. On the Estimation of Lorenz Curves from Grouped Observations. *Int Econ Rev* 1973;**14**:278-92.

115. Wagstaff A. The bounds of the concentration index when the variable of interest is binary, with an application to immunization inequality. *Health Econ* 2005;**14**:429-32.

116. Clarke PM, Gerdtham UG, Johannesson M, Bingefors K, Smith L. On the measurement of relative and absolute income-related health inequality. *Soc Sci Med* 2002;**55**:1923-28.

117. Wagstaff A, van Doorslaer E, Watanabe N. On Decomposing the Causes of Health Sector Inequalities with an Application to Malnutrition Inequalities in Vietnam. *J Econometrics* 2003;**112**:207-23.

118. Chen CN, Tsaur TW, Rhai TS. The Gini Coefficient and Negative Income. *Oxford Econ Papers* 1982;**34**:473-78.

119. Wagstaff A. Inequality aversion, health inequalities and health achievement. *J Health Econ* 2002;**21**:627-41.

120. Manor O, Matthews S, Power C. Comparing measures of health inequality. *Soc Sci Med* 1997;**45**:761-71.

121. Schneider MC, Castillo-Salgado C, Bacallao J, Loyola E, Mujica OJ, Vidaurre M, Roca A. Methods for measuring health inequalities (Part II). *Epidemiol Bull* 2005;**26**:5-10.

122. Pappa E, Niakas D. Assessment of health care needs and utilization in a mixed public-private system: the case of the Athens area. *BMC Health Serv Res* 2006;**6**:146

123. Gravelle H, Sutton M. Income related inequalities in self assessed health in Britain: 1979-1995. *J Epidemiol Community Health* 2003;**57**:125-29.

124. van Doorslaer E, Koolman X, Jones AM. Explaining income-related inequalities in doctor utilisation in Europe. *Health Econ* 2004;**13**:629-47.

125. Lu JR, Leung GM, Kwon S, Tin KYK, van Doorslaer E, O'Donnell O. Horizontal equity in health care utilization evidence from three high-income Asian economies. *Soc Sci Med* 2007;**64**:199-212.

126. Petersen PE, Kjøller M, Christensen LB, Krustrup U. Voksenbefolkningens tandstatus og udnyttelse af tandplejetilbuddet i Danmark 2000: Sociale og adfærdsmæssige determinanter for udvikling [Adult dental health status and use of oral health services in Denmark 2000. Sociobehavioural

determinants for improvement in oral health]. *Tandlaegebladet.* 2003;**107**:672-84.

127. Vallgårda S, Krasnik A, Vrangbæk K. Health Care Systems in Transition: Denmark. Thomson, S. and Mossialos, E. 2001. *European Observatory on Health Care Systems. Health Care Systems in Transition.*

128. Vrangbæk K, Christiansen T. Health Policy in Denmark: Leaving the Decentralized Welfare Path? *J Health Politics, Policy and Law* 2005;**30**:29-52.

129. Pedersen KM, Christiansen T, Bech M. The Danish health care system: evolution - not revolution - in a decentralized system. *Health Econ* 2005;**14**:S41-S57.

130. Gundgaard J, Søndergaard B. *Maskinel dosisdispensering i det primære sundhedsvæsen: Analyse af registerdata* [Dose Dispensing Medicine in the Primary Health Care Sector: A Register Based Study]. 2005. CAST, University of Southern Denmark; The Danish University of Pharmaceutical Sciences; Pharmakon.

131. Retsinformation. *Sundhedsloven: LOV nr 546 af 24/06/2005* [The Health Law]. 2005.

132. The Ministry of Interior and Health. *Sund hele livet - de nationale mål og strategier for folkesundheden 2002-10* [The Danish Government Programme on Public Health and Health Promotion]. 2002. Schultz Information.

133. Ministry of Health. *Regeringens folkesundhedsprogram 1999-2008: Et handlingsorienteret progam for sundere rammer i hverdagen* [The Danish Government Programme on Public Health and Health Promotion]. 1999.

134. Vallgarda S. Governing people's lives. Strategies for improving the health of the nations in England, Denmark, Norway and Sweden. *Eur J Public Health* 2001;**11**:386-92.

135. Statistics Denmark. StatBank Denmark, BEF1. www.dst.dk. 2007.

136. Ministry of Interior and Health. *Sundhedssektoren i tal - 2001/2002* [The Health Care Sector in Numbers – 2001/2002]. 2002.

137. Fyns Amt. Sundhedsplan 2000: *Forebyggelsesstrategi* [Health Plan 2000: Prevention Strategy]. 2007. Fyns Amt.

138. Gundgaard J, Sørensen J. *Evaluering af Fyns Amts Forebyggelsesstrategi: Baseline survey om sundhedstilstand og adfærd omkring tobak, alkohol, kost og motion* [Evaluation of the Prevention Strategy in Funen County: Baseline Survey on Behaviour with respect to Tobacco, Alcohol, Diet and Exercise]. 2002. Odense, CAST, University of Southern Denmark.

139. Sektionen för Surveystatistik and Svenska statistikersamfundet. Standard for bortfallsberäkning [Standard for calculating non-response]. 2005.

140. Elliott MN, Edwards C, Angeles J, Hambarsoomians K, Hays RD. Patterns of Unit and Item Nonresponse in the CAHPS Hospital Survey. *Health Serv Res* 2005;**40**:2096-119.

141. Jay GM, Liang J, Liu X, Sugisawa H. Patterns of nonresponse in a national survey of elderly Japanese. *J Gerontol* 1993;**48**:S143-S152.

142. Korkeila K, Suominen S, Ahvenainen J, Ojanlatva A, Rautava P, Helenius H, Koskenvuo M. Non-response and related factors in a nation-wide health survey. *Eur J Epidemiol* 2001;**17**:991-99.

143. Lamers LM. Medical consumption of respondents and non-respondents to a mailed health survey. *Eur J Public Health* 1997;**7**:267-71.

144. Sogaard AJ, Selmer R, Bjertness E, Thelle D. The Oslo Health Study: The impact of self-selection in a large, population-based survey. *Int J Equity Health* 2004;**3**:3.

145. Helasoja V, Prattala R, Dregval L, Pudule I, Kasmel A. Late response and item nonresponse in the Finbalt Health Monitor survey. *Eur J Public Health* 2002;**12**:117-23.

146. van den Akker M, Buntinx F, Metsemakers JF, Knottnerus JA. Morbidity in responders and non-responders in a register-based population survey. *Fam Pract* 1998;**15**:261-63.

147. Ministry of Interior and Health – National Board of Health. *Takstsystem 2003 – Vejledning* [System of Charges - Manual]. National Board of Health, 2002.

148. Hallas J, Hansen NC. Individual utilization of anti-asthma medication by young adults: a prescription database analysis. *J Intern Med* 1993;**234**:65-70.

149. Hallas J. Conducting pharmacoepidemiologic research in Denmark. *Pharmacoepidemiol Drug Saf* 2001;**10**:619-23.

150. Danish Medicines Agency. *Lægemiddelstatistik 1997-2001 Danmark: Den primære sundhedssektor. Sygehussektoren* [Medicinal Product Statistics 1997-2001: The primary health care sector. The hospital sector]. Danish Medicines Agency, 2002.

151. Odense Universitetshospital and Sygehus Fyn. *2001 årsberetning* [Annual Report 2001]. 2002.

152. National Board of Health. *Sygehusenes virksomhed 2002 (foreløbig opgørelse)*. [Hospital Activity (provisional status)] Årgang 6, nr. 9. 2002. Nye tal fra Sundhedsstyrelsen.

153. Statistics Denmark. StatBank Denmark, PRIS6. www.dst.dk. 2006. 28-10-2003.

154. Brooks R. EuroQol: the current state of play. *Health Policy* 1996;**37**:53-72.

155. Dolan P. Modeling valuations for EuroQol health states. *Med Care* 1997;**35**:1095-108.

156. The EuroQol Group. EuroQol--a new facility for the measurement of health-related quality of life. *Health Policy* 1990;**16**:199-208.

157. Dolan P. The Measurement of Health-Related Quality of Life for Use in Resource Allocation Decisions in Health Care. *Handbook of health economics. Volume 1B* 2000;1723-60.

158. Drummond MF, O'Brien B, Stoddart GL, Torrance GW. *Methods for the Economic Evaluation of Health Care Programmes*. Second Edition ed. Oxford University Press, 1997.

159. Pedersen KM, Wittrup-Jensen KU, Brooks R, Gudex C. *Værdisætning af sundhed: Teorien om kvalitetsjusterede leveår og en dansk anvendelse*. Odense: Syddansk Universitetsforlag, 2003.

160. Wittrup-Jensen KU, Lauridsen JT, Gudex C, Brooks R, and Pedersen KM. Estimating danish EQ-5D tariffs using the time trade-off (TTO) and visual analogue scale (VAS) methods. In Norinder AL, Pedersen KM, Roos P (eds) *Proceedings of the 18th*

Plenary Meeting of the EuroQol Group, 6th - 7th September, 2001, Copenhagen, Denmark, IHE- The Swedish Institute for Health Economics, Lund. 2001.

161. Bjørner JB, Damsgaard MT, Watt T, Groenvold M. Tests of data quality, scaling assumptions, and reliability of the Danish SF-36. *J Clin Epidemiol* 1998;**51**:1001-11.

162. Brazier J. The SF-36 health survey questionnaire--a tool for economists. *Health Econ* 1993;**2**:213-15.

163. Yost KJ, Haan MN, Levine RA, Gold EB. Comparing SF-36 scores across three groups of women with different health profiles. *Qual Life Res* 2005;**14**:1251-61.

164. Bjørner JB, Damsgaard MT, Watt T, Bech P, Rasmussen NK, Kristensen TS, Modvig J, Thunedborg K. Dansk manual til SF-36 [Danish Manual for SF-36]. Lif Lægemiddelindustriforeningen, 1997.

165. Ware JE, Gandek B, Kosinski M, Aaronson NK, Apolone G, Brazier J, Bullinger M, Kaasa S, Leplege A, Prieto L, Sullivan M, Thunedborg K. The equivalence of SF-36 summary health scores estimated using standard and country-specific algorithms in 10 countries: Results from the IQOLA Project. *Journal of Clinical Epidemiology* 1998;**51**:1167-70.

166. Lynch J, Kaplan G. Socioeconomic Position. In: Berkman LF, Kawachi I, editors. *Social Epidemiology*. New York: Oxford University Press, 2000:13-35.

Chapter 2

Income related inequality in prescription drugs in Denmark

Jens Gundgaard

Pharmacoepidemiology and Drug Safety 2005; 14: 307-317

Summary

Purpose: To examine income-related inequity in utilisation of prescription drugs in Funen County, Denmark after a new reimbursement system was implemented.

Methods: An individual level prescription database was merged with a health survey of 2,927 respondents interviewed in 2000 and 2001 about their health status and socio-economic and socio-demographic characteristics. An index of horizontal inequity was used to estimate the degree of inequity in drug utilisation across income groups, using the indirect method of standardisation to control for age, gender and health status as a proxy for need. The results were compared to estimates from a traditional regression analysis.

Results: The least advantaged with respect to income consume a bigger share of the prescription drugs than the most advantaged. After standardisation for age, gender and health status the least advantaged have a lower share of the drug consumption than expected. However, traditional regression analysis showed no signs of an income effect on the level of consumption of prescription drugs.

Conclusion: The index of horizontal inequity suggests that some horizontal inequity favouring the better off is present. However, the results deviate from what can be found by traditional regression analysis.

Key words: prescription drugs, prescription database, utilisation, inequality, inequity, concentration index, standardisation

Introduction

Equal access to health care across socio-economic groups is one of the main objectives of health policy.[1-3] The concentration index has become a standard method for measuring income related inequalities in health and health care utilisation.[4-9] The concentration index is a generalised Gini coefficient and is a measure of how equal one variable is distributed with respect to the ranking of another variable.[10] Concentration indices have been used to measure socio-economic inequalities in hospital utilisation, physician and medical specialist visits.[8] However, the concentration index has not been used to describe utilisation of prescription drugs.

Total sales of partly or fully reimbursed drugs amounted to DKK 1430 per capita in 2001 in Denmark.[11] This is a considerable fraction of total health care expenditures (close to 10% of the overall health care expenditures.[12] In Denmark, health care is mainly financed through general taxation. However, for dentistry, physiotherapy and medicine a high degree of co-payment exists.[13] In the spring of 2000, a new reimbursement system for prescription drugs was implemented. Before the new system was implemented a proportional subsidy was given to a list of drugs, that were entitled to subsidy, regardless the level of consumption of the individual consumer. After the implementation, the subsidies follow the individual at a progressive rate, such that a higher percentage is given to large-scale consumers of prescription drugs.

The association between socio-economic status and medicine use is not yet clear, as various studies vary in methodology, definitions of socio-economic status or focus on specific pharmaceutical groups. Given the difficulty of gathering individual level data on drug consumption a number of studies have been ecological. An ecological Swedish study about utilisation of major drug groups in an urban Swedish population reported a negative correlation between drug consumption and income (significant for males only).[14] A population-based Canadian study reported that the highest use of pharmaceuticals is found in the lower income quintiles and in areas with greatest socio-economic risks.[15] Another Canadian study found that the per capita total drug expenditures in the 1980s were considerably higher in low-income families compared to high-income families. The study was undertaken to determine whether drug programmes were successful in reducing out-of-pocket pharmaceutical expenditure for low-income families.[16]

Individual based studies have also been carried out. A Norwegian health survey examined the drug pattern in the general population during a two-week period and used education as a socio-economic status variable. The study showed increasing drug use with decreasing levels of education, but after adjusting for morbidity high education became a weak predictor for drug use.[17] In another Norwegian health survey education was also found to have only minor importance when adjusting for morbidity.[18] A Dutch study about the socio-economic differences in the utilisation of health services in the Netherlands showed higher utilisation rates of prescription medicine for lower educational groups compared to those with an academic background. Controlling for socio-demographic background variables and health status, the differences diminished or reversed the relationship across educational groups.[19] According to the Danish Health and Morbidity Survey the consumption of prescription drugs follows the pattern of illness such that people with less education use prescription drugs more regularly compared to people with more education. That is, people with lower socio-economic status do not seem to have less access to pharmaceuticals in Denmark.[20]

If utilisation of medicine varies with socio-economic status like income even after controlling for socio-demographic characteristics like age and gender, and the need for medicine, the distribution and use of medicine in the population might not be rational. Furthermore, it would be considered inequitable if use of medicine was systematically related to characteristics like socio-economic status when need is controlled for.[21]

In this study, survey data on health status and socio-economic status have been merged with an individual level prescription database, and concentration indices are used to measure to what extent socio-economic inequalities in prescription drugs exist in Denmark after the implementation of the new reimbursement system. The results are compared to estimates from traditional regression analysis.

Material and methods

Data collection

The data set used for the analysis is a combination of survey data and an individual level prescription database. Five-thousand people living in Funen County, Denmark aged 16-80 were drawn from The Centralised Civil Register to participate in a health survey on health status, health behaviour and socio-economic background. The sample was stratified with respect to municipalities, such that small and large municipalities would be represented. Within municipalities the respondents were drawn randomly. Funen County is situated right in the middle of Denmark and the county population makes up a little less than 10% of the national population, and is considered representative of the Danes in many respects.[20] The data were gathered through telephone interviews that took place in the period from October 2000 through April 2001.[22]

The survey data were merged with data from Odense University Pharmacoepidemiologic Database (OPED). This database consists of individual level data on all prescription refunds from Funen County. Each purchase of reimbursed drugs from a pharmacy in Funen County is described by brand name of the drug, dose unit, quantity and date of prescription.[23] About 75% of all medicine sold outside hospitals are reimbursed medicine.[11] The database does not contain information on over-the-counter-medicine (e.g. salicylates, acetaminophene, ibuprofen, some ulcer drugs, antihistamines, and laxatives). Furthermore, prescription drugs not entitled to reimbursement are not included in the database either (oral contraceptives, benzodiazepines, and certain antibiotics).[24] The prescription data were drawn from the database for the years 2000 and 2001. In addition, the purchases included in the study were limited to after 1 March 2000 as this was the day the new reimbursement system was implemented in Denmark.

Variables

Table 1 includes a list of variables used in the study. Drug consumption is measured in two ways. The first one is using the concept of defined daily dose (DDD), which is the recommended average dose for a particular drug per 24 hours for an adult who takes the medicine for its main indication.[11] For each individual in the study the number of DDDs is summed over the 22 months period. The other way of measuring the quantity of drug consumption is in monetary units using the total sales per person during the 22 months period measured in pharmacy retail prices. The pharmacy retail prices change every 2 weeks and have therefore been adjusted according to the monthly CPI in Denmark. The two different ways of measuring drug consumption might give different results as people, who are heavy users in terms of DDD, might not necessarily be the same people who use the most expensive drugs.

Socio-economic status is included as gross income the previous year taken from the health survey. The income is a categorical variable consisting of 17 intervals. The sample population is ranked according to the categories. Within each category the respondents are ordered randomly.

Age and gender are measured by a dummy variable for being female from the health survey and a continuous variable for age from the The Centralised Civil Register. Age is taken to the power of two and three making it possible to carry out polynomial regression.

Health status is included as a proxy for need. Two variables are used. One variable consists of EuroQol utilities, which is a continuous variable with values on a scale from 1 (perfect health) to 0 (death).[25-27] Negative values are allowed for health states worse than death. Danish *Time Trade Off* weights were used to calculate the utilities.[28] The other measure is a dummy vector with categorical answers to a question about general health. The categories can be seen in Table 1.

Predicting consumption of prescription drugs

Regression analysis is carried out to standardise the consumption of prescription drugs. It is assumed that each individual's need for medicine can be characterised by the mean level of medicine for people with the same age, gender and health status.[8] As is normal for cost data or data for utilisation of health care, consumption of prescription drugs is badly skewed to the right.[29,30] That is, a few people have a large level of consumption whereas most people have a small level of consumption. A considerable fraction of the population does not have any consumption at all, which exacerbates the skewness and complicates the estimation procedures.

Tabel 1. Variable list

Variable group	Variable name	Explanation
Dependent variables	DDD	Prescription drug consumption measured in DDD[†]
	DKK	Prescription drug consumption measured in expenditure, DKK[‡]
SES*	INCOME	Annual gross income
Age and gender	FEMALE	Dummy variable: Female=1, Male=0
	AGE	Age
	AGE2	Age to the power of 2
	AGE3	Age to the power of 3
Need proxies	EQUTILITY	EuroQol-5D utility, Danish TTO weights
	EXCELLENT	General health: Excellent
	VERYGOOD	General health: Very good
	GOOD	General health: Good
	FAIR	General health: Fair
	POOR	General health: Poor

* SES = Socio-economic status.
[†] DDD = Defined daily dose.
[‡] DKK = Denmark Kroner.

To tackle the problem generated by the zero-consumption observations, a two-part regression model (TPM) is used to predict the level of medicine consumption for each individual. The TPM consists of a logistic regression model to predict the probability of having non-zero consumption (part 1), and a semi-log linear regression model to predict the level of consumption given non-zero consumption (part 2). The dependent variable is log transformed to remove the skewness of the distribution.[30] The predicted values of log consumption are then retransformed using the so-called smearing estimator to convert the predicted consumption back into the original scale. The predicted level of consumption is:

$$E(m_i|X) = \Pr(m_i > 0|X) \, e^{X\beta} S \qquad (1)$$

where the probability function is the first part of the TPM, m_i is medicine consumption of the ith individual, $e^{X\beta}$ is the exponentiated expected value on the log-scale of the linear regression with the vector X of explanatory variables and S is the smearing estimator, which is the average of the exponentiated residuals.[30,31]

The advantage of using a TPM is that the probability of consuming prescription drugs and the level of prescription drugs consumed for consumers are described by different functions as it is most likely not the same mechanisms that determine the barriers of starting to consume as the amount of prescription drugs consumed for people who are already consumers.

The index of horizontal inequity

The degree of income related inequality in consumption of prescription drugs is quantified by the index of horizontal inequity (HI_{WV}), which is based on concentration indices, and includes standardisation for relevant need-based variables. As described in van Doorslaer *et al.* and Kakwani *et al.* a concentration curve for drug consumption is the cumulative proportion of drug use as a function of the cumulative proportion of the population ranked by socio-economic status (in this case income).[6,8] The concentration curve is illustrated in Figure 1 and denoted $L_M(R)$, where R is the relative rank. The concentration curve is expected to be concave towards the origin, as the disadvantaged groups (with respect to socio-economic status) tend to have a relatively higher consumption of medicine. Quantification of inequality is done by the concentration index C_M, which is twice the area between $L_M(R)$ and the 45° line in Figure 1. The concentration index can be calculated by the formula:

$$C_M = \frac{2}{Nm} \sum_{i=1}^{N} m_i R_i - 1 \qquad (2)$$

where N is the sample size, m_i is medicine consumption of the ith individual, m is the mean medicine consumption and R_i is the fractional rank of the ith individual with respect to income. The concentration index ranges between -1 and 1. If the concentration curve is concave C_M

will have a negative sign, indicating inequality in favour of the most disadvantaged, and C_M will have a positive sign if the concentration curve is convex, indicating inequality in favour of the better off (see Box 1).

Figure 1. Example of concentration curves

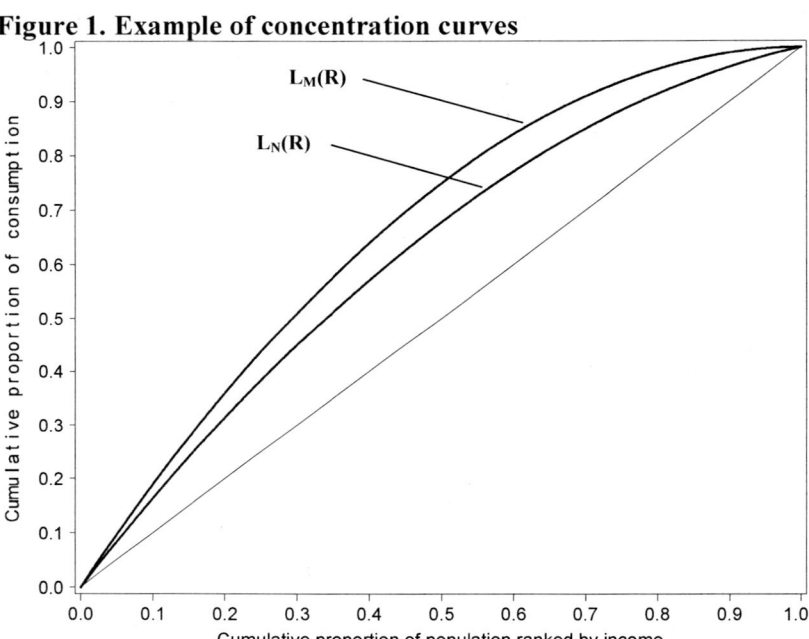

$L_m(R)$ = Observed concentration curve
$L_n(R)$ = Concentration curve for need

The concentration index is only appropriate as long as individuals are expected to have the same level of consumption, that is, a distribution that follows the 45° line in Figure 1. However, older people and people with health problems are expected to be in higher need of drug consumption, and a higher level of consumption among those groups will seldom be characterised as inequitable. Consequently, the distribution of actual consumption should be compared to what could be expected due to variation in need (predicted consumption from the TPM). The predicted consumption can be obtained by indirect standardisation of the consumption. The quantification of inequality can be standardised indirectly by predicting the expected level of consumption m_i^* for the individual given age, gender and health status which works as a proxy for need. By using the indirect standardisation method, it is assumed that individuals at a given income level will have the same consumption as the rest of the population when adjusting for age, gender and health status. A concentration curve for predicted consumption $L_N(R)$ is illustrated in Figure 1, and the predicted inequality can be calculated using Equation 2 with replacement of m and m_i with m^* and m_i^*, respectively:

$$C_N = \frac{2}{Nm^*} \sum_{i=1}^{N} m_i^* R_i - 1. \tag{3}$$

For calculating the index of horizontal inequity the concentration curve $L_M(R)$ is compared with $L_N(R)$ as opposed to the 45° line or:

$$HI_{WV} = C_M - C_N. \tag{4}$$

A non-zero value of the HI_{WV} index implies that the actual distribution does not follow the distribution of need, and people in equal need are not treated equally. A positive value indicates inequity in favour of the higher income groups (Box 1). There are several methods of quantifying inequalities.[32,33] Compared to other indices the HI_{WV} index has some advantages that are worth mentioning: (1) The inequalities in medicine consumption are analysed with respect to socio-economic status. In this analysis income is used. (2) The measure includes the whole sampled population, not just the lower and upper income groups. (3) The index is sensitive to changes in the distribution of the population across income groups. (4) The index can be illustrated graphically (as in Figure 1). (5) The index can be tested for statistical significance.[7] The latter can be done by regression analysis. If the relative consumption multiplied by twice the variance of the relative rank is regressed on the relative rank, then the OLS coefficient of the relative rank is the concentration index C_M:

$$2\sigma_R^2 \frac{m_i}{m} = \alpha + C_M R_i + u_i, \tag{5}$$

and standard errors and t-values are easily obtained from standard statistical packages. The standard errors for the HI_{WV} index are not easily obtained, as C_M and C_N are not independently distributed. However, they can be obtained by including the observed relative consumption and the predicted relative consumption on the left-hand side of the regression:

$$2\sigma_R^2\left[\frac{m_i}{m} - \frac{m_i^*}{m^*}\right] = \alpha + HI_{WV} R_i + u_i. \tag{6}$$

The OLS estimator for the coefficient of the relative rank is then the HI_{WV} index. However, the standard errors are only an approximation to the real standard errors as the residuals per definition are serially correlated.[6,8]

Box 1. Interpretation of the concentration index and horizontal inequity index

A positive value of C_M indicates an unequal distribution in favour of the higher income groups.
A negative value of C_M indicates an unequal distribution in favour of the lower income groups.
A zero index value of C_M indicates an equal distribution.
A positive value of HI_{WV} indicates horizontal inequity in favour of the higher income groups.
A negative value of HI_{WV} indicates horizontal inequity in favour of the lower income groups.
A zero index value of HI_{WV} indicates no horizontal inequity (or crossing concentration curves).

Inequality estimates from traditional regression analysis

Another and more traditional way to investigate inequality, than using concentration indices, is to include the socio-economic status variable, income, directly into a regression model. A significant coefficient for this variable, controlling for age, gender and health status, indicates that income affects the level of consumption.[19,34] To explore this approach, and to compare it with the HI_{WV} index, a separate TPM is estimated where continuous income (approximated by the midpoints of the intervals) is added to the model.

Results

Study population

Due to non-response not all 5,000 people, who were invited to participate, did participate. Table 2 is a frequency table of the number of people who participated in the study and the number of people who didn't participate for various reasons. 1578 (31.6%) people were not interviewed for the health survey as they refused to participate, were not found, or were not able to participate for some other reason. This leaves us with a survey of 3422 (68.4%) respondents. However, not all the respondents answered all the relevant questions and had to be excluded from the study. As is typical, income is the sensitive question that people abstain from answering. The final working sample is thus 2927 respondents with a response rate of 59%. Table 3 shows descriptive statistics for the relevant variables. For income the descriptive statistics is calculated using midpoints of the intervals.

A response/non-response analysis has been carried out using logistic regression for participating in the working sample. The analyses show that participation is a slightly non-linear function of age with the middle-aged being the most prone to participate. Gender is not significant. Being a consumer of medicine does not seem to be of importance for responding or not responding in the survey, whereas the level of consumption measured by DDD does have a negative impact on the likelihood of participating. The analysis indicates that the consumption of prescription drugs is more skewed among the non-respondents. Presumably a group of people is missing from the survey due to bad health and is expected to have a higher level of consumption of medicine, than what we see among the respondents.

Tabel 2. Response and non-response

Participation status	Reason	Frequency	%
Response	Participate	2927	58.54
Internal non-response	Income missing	483	9.66
	Health status missing	9	0.18
	Income and health status missing	2	0.04
	Other	1	0.02
External non-response	Refuse to participate	996	19.92
	Not found	273	5.46
	Other	309	6.18

Inequality estimates

The results from a two-part model used for one of the standardisation procedures are presented in Table 4. The two parts of the model include the same explanatory variables, that is, a dummy for gender, a polynomial function of age, and a EuroQol utility. Twenty-eight percent of the respondents were not consumers over the 22 months period. The two-part model indicates that women have twice the odds of being consumers compared to men (OR=2.0480), and among people who are already consumers women consume 34% more prescription drugs than men (coef=0.3413). Age is taken to the power of two in the logistic model, whereas it is taken to the power of three in the linear regression. The chance of being consumers and the level of consumption increase with age, and is fit well by polynomial regression. As a proxy for need the coefficient for the utility variable is negative in the two parts indicating increasing consumption at lower health status. An increase in the utility score by 0.01 decreases the odds of being a consumer by 3% (OR=$0.0430^{1/100}$), and given non-zero consumption an increase in the utility score by 0.01 decreases consumption by 2% (coef=-2.0190). Using a TPM to solve the zero consumption problem and a semilog model to diminish the skew makes the residuals approximately normally distributed. In Table 5 the two-part model has been repeated with the general health dummy vector as opposed to the EuroQol utility variable. The reference dummy is poor general health. The change in variables for health status does not have a big impact on the models' conclusions. As expected, the better the general health state is, the smaller is the chance of being a consumer or have a high level of consumption. The two standardisation procedures have been repeated for expenditures instead of DDD. These models show similar results and are therefore not shown.

The HI_{WV} index is depicted graphically in Figure 2. It is shown for inequality in prescription drugs measured in DDDs and standardised with age, gender, and EuroQol utilities. The $L_M(R)$-curve is concave showing that the least advantaged with respect to income have the highest share of the medicine consumption. An exception is the income group of the first two deciles, where the $L_M(R)$-curve is below the 45° line. This group of people is younger than the average and has a large fraction of people in the educational system. The $L_N(R)$-curve lies above the he $L_M(R)$-curve indicating that even though the least advantaged have the highest share of the consumption it is not as high as expected. As can be seen in Table 6 the HI_{WV} index is 0.10 and significant demonstrating inequity favouring the better off. It is of little importance which health variable is used.

Table 3. Descriptive statistics for working sample (N=2927)

Variable	Min	Max	Mean	Median	SD
Annual income*, DKK[†]	0	774500	202218	174500	128083
EQ-utility	-0.27	1	0.90	1	0.15
Number of expeditions	0	192	8.99	2	17.28
DDD[‡]	0	8054	389	30	841
Expenditures, DKK	0	79189	2216	229	5244
Consumer	0	1	0.74	1	0.44
Female	0	1	0.49	0	0.50
Age	16	80	44.67	44	16.23

* Interval midpoints.
[‡] DDD = Defined daily dose.
[†] DKK = Denmark Kroner.

The calculations have been repeated with consumption of prescription drugs measured in expenditures using pharmacy retail prices. The HI_{WV} index coefficient is a little bit bigger when using expenditures. However, the difference is not noteworthy, and the distribution of expenditures seems to follow the distribution of DDDs.

Table 7 shows a TPM equivalent to Table 4 but where income is added to the model. The coefficients are close to zero in the two parts and none of the coefficients are statistically significant different from zero. According to this method, controlling for age, gender and health status, income does not have an influence on the probability or the level of consumption indicating no horizontal inequity.

Discussion

A new reimbursement system was implemented in Denmark to create a more equitable system, such that the consumers will get reimbursed according to the amount of medicine consumed and not according to the type of medicine consumed. In addition, the reimbursement increases at a progressive rate to secure that need is the first and foremost determining factor for the amount consumed. The system does work in the sense that the least advantaged with respect to income, who are also the most needy, consume a bigger share of the medicine than the well-off. The question is whether they consume as much as they could be expected to do. The HI_{WV} index suggests that this is not the case, assuming the average level of consumption given age, gender and health status is the appropriate level. This assumption, however, might not necessarily be correct, e.g. some socio-economic groups might use more medicine than what can be considered to be rational.

Figure 2. Concentration curves for actual and expected medicine consumption in DDD

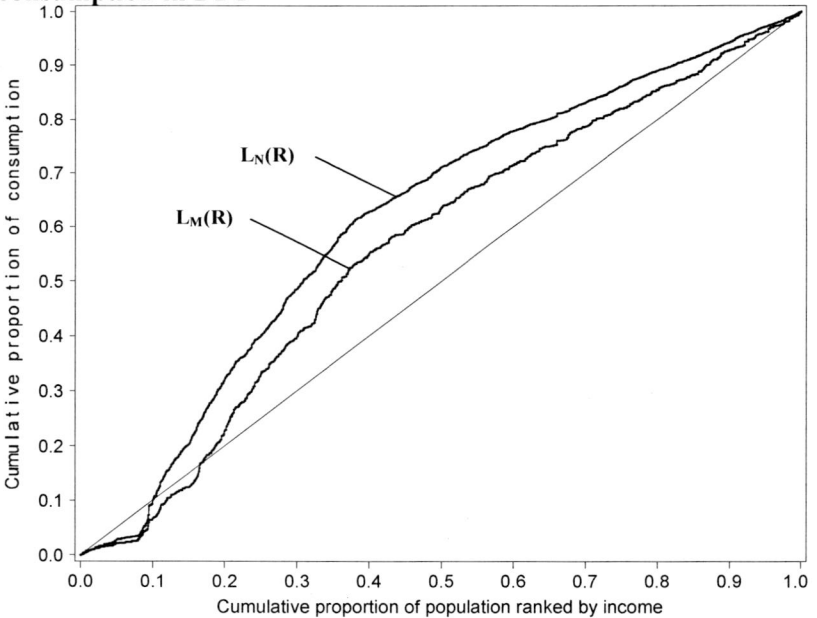

$L_m(R)$ = Observed concentration curve
$L_n(R)$ = Concentration curve for expected medicine consumption

Table 4. Two-part model for consumption of prescription drugs measured in DDD

Part 1: Logistic regression						Part 2: Semilog regression				
Variable	Coef	SE	Chi-Square	p-value	OR	Variable	Coef	SE	t-value	p-value
INTERCEPT	3.3863	0.4950	46.81	<.0001	29.5560	INTERCEPT	6.9284	0.6700	10.34	<.0001
FEMALE	0.7168	0.0877	66.86	<.0001	2.0480	FEMALE	0.3413	0.0712	4.79	<.0001
AGE	-0.0210	0.0153	1.89	0.1696	0.9790	AGE	-0.1765	0.0467	-3.78	0.0002
AGE2	0.0005	0.0002	8.12	0.0044	1.0005	AGE2	0.0050	0.0011	4.74	<.0001
EQUTILITY	-3.1406	0.3840	66.91	<.0001	0.0430	AGE3	0.0000	<.0001	-4.41	<.0001
						EQUTILITY	-2.0190	0.2157	-9.36	<.0001
Observations	2927					Observations	2114			
Positive consumption	2114					F-value	189.03			
Zero consumption	813					p-value	<.0001			
Likelihood Ratio test:						R-Square	0.3096			
Chi-square	257.95					Smearing factor	3.072			
p-value	<.0001									

Tabel 5. Two-part model for consumption of prescription drugs measured in DDD

Part 1: Logistic regression						Part 2: Semilog regression				
Variable	Coef	SE	Chi-Square	p-value	OR	Variable	Coef	SE	t-value	p-value
INTERCEPT	2.4325	0.6785	12.85	0.0003	11.3870	INTERCEPT	6.3987	0.6544	9.78	<.0001
FEMALE	0.7593	0.0882	74.14	<.0001	2.1370	FEMALE	0.3490	0.0698	5.00	<.0001
AGE	-0.0163	0.0154	1.13	0.2881	0.9840	AGE	-0.1511	0.0458	-3.30	0.0010
AGE2	0.0004	0.0002	5.19	0.0227	1.0000	AGE2	0.0044	0.0010	4.21	<.0001
EXCELLENT	-2.5149	0.6013	17.49	<.0001	0.0810	AGE3	0.0000	0.0000	-3.92	<.0001
VERYGOOD	-2.1867	0.5975	13.39	0.0003	0.1120	EXCELLENT	-2.0999	0.2212	-9.49	<.0001
GOOD	-1.6491	0.5976	7.62	0.0058	0.1920	VERYGOOD	-1.7352	0.2087	-8.31	<.0001
FAIR	-0.6709	0.6401	1.10	0.2946	0.5110	GOOD	-1.3776	0.2052	-6.71	<.0001
						FAIR	-0.5288	0.2251	-2.35	0.0189
Observations	2927					Observations	2114			
Positive consumption	2114					F-value	134.68			
Zero consumption	813					p-value	<.0001			
Likelihood Ratio test:						R-Square	0.3386			
Chi-square	293.68					Smearing factor	2.887			
p-value	<.0001									

Table 6. Concentration indices and HI indices

Unit	Need proxy	C_M*	SE[‡]	t-value	p-value	HI[†]	SE[‡]	t-value	p-value
DDD[§]	EQ-5D Utility	-0.1311	0.0229	-5.72	<.0001	0.1032	0.0218	4.73	<.0001
	Health variable	-0.1311	0.0229	-5.72	<.0001	0.1076	0.0208	5.17	<.0001
DKK[¶]	EQ-5D Utility	-0.1022	0.0252	-4.06	<.0001	0.1126	0.0245	4.60	<.0001
	Health variable	-0.1022	0.0252	-4.06	<.0001	0.1142	0.0232	4.92	<.0001

*C_M = Observed concentration index
[†] HI = Index of horizontal inequity.
[‡] SE = Standard Error.
[§] DDD = Defined daily dose.
[¶] DKK = Denmark Kroner.

Tabel 7. Two-part model for consumption of prescription drugs measured in DDD (income included)

Part 1: Logistic regression						Part 2: Semilog regression				
Variable	Coef	SE	Chi-Square	p-value	OR	Variable	Coef	SE	t-value	p-value
INTERCEPT	3.5684	0.5185	47.36	<.0001	35.4610	INTERCEPT	6.6396	0.6967	9.53	<.0001
FEMALE	0.7546	0.0931	65.74	<.0001	2.1270	FEMALE	0.3019	0.0759	3.98	<.0001
AGE	-0.0331	0.0183	3.27	0.0707	0.9670	AGE	-0.1540	0.0490	-3.14	0.0017
AGE2	0.0006	0.0002	9.31	0.0023	1.0010	AGE2	0.0046	0.0011	4.25	<.0001
EQUTILITY	-3.1971	0.3870	68.24	<.0001	0.0410	AGE3	0.0000	<.0001	-4.09	<.0001
INCOME	0.0000	<.0001	1.46	0.2274	1.0000	EQUTILITY	-1.9710	0.2179	-9.04	<.0001
						INCOME	0.0000	<.0001	-1.51	0.1323
Observations	2927					Observations	2114			
Positive consumption	2114					F-value	157.99			
Zero consumption	813					p-value	<.0001			
Likelihood Ratio test:						R-Square	0.3103			
Chi-square	259.42					Smearing factor	3.066			
p-value	<.0001									

The combination of survey data and computerised registers has advantages and drawbacks. Computerised registers are most often more precise, include a long history, and are accessible for a large number of observations. Survey data are often characterised by missing observations, recall bias and a limited number of observations. However, surveys make it possible to gather data that are not available through registries (e.g. self perceived health). In this study the combination of survey data and computerised registers made it possible to standardise individual consumption of prescription drugs retrieved from a computerised register with age, gender and self-assessed health status. The sample size was 5,000 individuals. Yet, due to external and internal non-response the final working sample was a little less than 3,000 individuals. This is still enough to be representative for the Danish population if there is no non-response bias. But the non-response analysis suggested that the non-respondents had a higher level of drug consumption than respondents, even though they were not more likely to be consumers during the period of analysis. It is always a problem for the validity of the study when the risk of non-response is correlated with a variable of interest.

The survey data were gathered through telephone interviews. This means that people too weak to carry through a telephone conversation obviously are not included in the study. This could be one explanation for the higher level of medicine consumption among the non-respondents. Although it is known that the non-respondents have a higher level of consumption of prescription drugs, it is not easy to speculate on the effect on the results. Less non-response will most likely lead to a higher index value of C_M. The value of the HI_{WV} index, however, depends on consumption compared to need, and need is unknown amongst the non-respondents.

The study covers only prescription medicine in the primary health care sector, and only prescription drugs entitled to reimbursement are in the database. In addition, prescription drugs bought from pharmacies outside Funen County, drugs used in hospitals and illegal purchases of drugs over the internet are not covered by the database either. To include more types of drugs in the study, it would have been necessary to add questions about drug consumption in the health survey.

The income variable was taken from the health survey. Income is a sensitive question and a large fraction of the respondents were reluctant to answer that question. Four hundred eighty-five respondents were left out of the analysis due to missing observations with respect to income. Presumably, people with a higher income are more reluctant to answer the income variable and this might have created another bias. Furthermore, the answers could be subject to recall bias, as not all people might remember their exact gross income from the previous year. On the other hand, the answers are given in income categories and the concentration indices might not be that sensitive to the precision of the income. In addition, the income variable was validated against official income statistics from the relevant year and there were no signs of considerable deviations. Still, an income variable from a computerised registry would have been preferred, or even better, a household income variable, as this type of income variable would have been a more valid variable for ability to pay. However, such variables were not available for the present study.

The medicine data were limited to the years 2000 and 2001. In addition, the first two months of the year 2000 were excluded as a new reimbursement system was implemented 1 March 2000. This amounts to a 22 months period. Medicine data were available for a longer period of time. The longer the period is, the smaller is the problem of zero consumption data and random fluctuations. However, the health status indicators are point estimates, and will be less valid as standardisation variables for consumption of prescription drugs taken place too long before or after the time of the interview. However, extending the period to 31 month did not lead to any substantial change in the results.

As a proxy for need for medicine consumption two measures for health status were used: EuroQol utilities and general self-assessed health. Health status as a proxy for need for health care services is common in the literature.[8,19,34] Health status is not always a good proxy for need for medicine. Some products are taken for the preventive effect. Furthermore, when medicine cures the illnesses the need for medicine is not accounted for by the health status indicators, which might show good or perfect health as a result of the medicine consumption. A more correct need indicator would be diagnoses for illnesses that induce need for medicine. However, these were not available for the present study. In addition, it would be a complicated task to make diagnoses operational in health surveys to solve the problem in question.

The analysis shows that the least advantaged with respect to income consume a bigger share of the prescription drugs than the most advantaged. This is in accordance with previous studies.[15-17,19,20] The consumption of prescription drugs is standardised with an indirect standardisation method. After standardisation for age, gender and health status the HI_{WV} index shows that the least advantaged have a lower share of the consumption than expected, and this suggests that some horizontal inequity favouring the better off is present. The indirect standardisation method has been carried out using a two-part model to predict each individual's level of consumption. The standardisation reverses the pattern of inequity in prescription drugs. Naturally, this causes some thoughtfulness. The two-part model seems to be in accordance with the idea that the probability of consumption and the level of consumption can be explained by two different mechanisms. In addition, the model seems to do fairly well with respect to regression diagnostics. Another way to investigate inequality is to include the socio-economic status variable directly in the standardising regression model. Using this traditional regression analysis no significant effect of income was found, indicating that income does not play an important role for the level of consumption. This naturally raises some doubts about the methodological robustness of the results from the HI_{WV} index. However, it is important to be aware of the fact that the two models measure different things. The regression approach measures the marginal effect of income on the level of consumption, whereas the HI_{WV} index measures how the distribution of consumption is related to the ranking of people according to income. The two approaches are not necessarily supposed to lead to the same conclusions. The HI_{WV} index was chosen as the preferred method, as concentration curves have become a standard method of measuring horizontal inequity, they have an intuitive interpretation and can be shown graphically. However, as the results deviate from what can be found by traditional regression analysis, it is up to the reader to decide how much weight the results should be given.

Conclusion

An individual level prescription database was merged with health survey data to analyse income related inequality in prescription drugs in Denmark after a new reimbursement system was implemented. The index of horizontal inequity was applied to estimate the degree of horizontal inequity. The analysis shows that the least advantaged with respect to income consume a bigger share of the prescription drugs than the most advantaged. The consumption of prescription drugs is standardised with an indirect standardisation method. After standardisation for age, gender and health status the least advantaged have a lower share of the consumption than expected, and this suggests that some horizontal inequity favouring the better off is present. However, the results differ from estimates from traditional regression analysis.

Acknowledgements

The study was carried out thanks to a research grant from The Health Insurance Foundation, Denmark.

KEY POINTS

- The lower income groups consume a bigger share of the total consumption of prescription drugs compared to the higher income groups measured in DDDs as well as monetary terms
- The lower income groups need more prescription drugs than the higher income groups according to age, gender and health status
- If consumption of prescription drugs does not follow the need distribution the consequence might be either over-utilisation or under-utilisation or horizontal inequity
- The reimbursement system, the level of co-payment, and socio-economic position may influence on the consumption of prescription drugs

References

1. The Copenhagen declaration on reducing social inequalities in health. *Scand J Public Health* 2002;**Suppl 59**:78-79.

2. Dahlgren G, Whitehead M. Policies and strategies to promote equity in health. 1-50. 2000. Copenhagen, WHO Regional Office for Europe.

3. Stronks G, Gunning-Schepers LJ. Should equity in health be target number 1. *Eur J Public Health* 1993;**65**:153-65.

4. Clarke PM, Gerdtham UG, Connelly LB. A note on the decomposition of the health concentration index. *Health Econ* 2003;**12**:511-16.

5. Humphries KH, van Doorslaer E. Income-related health inequality in Canada. *Soc Sci Med* 2000;**50**:663-71.

6. Kakwani N, Wagstaff A, van Doorslaer E. Socioeconomic Inequalities in Health: Measurement, Computation, and Statistical Inference. *J Econometrics* 1997;**77**:87-103.

7. van Doorslaer E, Wagstaff A, Bleichrodt H, Calonge S, Gerdtham UG, Gerfin, M, Geurts J, Gross L, Häkkinen U, Leu RE, O'Donnell O, Propper C, Puffer F, Rodríguez M, Sundberg G, Winkelhake O. Income-related inequalities in health: some international comparisons. *J Health Econ* 1997;**16**:93-112.

8. van Doorslaer E, Wagstaff A, van der Burg H, Christiansen T, De Graeve D, Duchesne I, Gerdtham UG, Gerfin M, Geurts J, Gross L, Häkkinen U, John J, Klavus J, Leu RE, Nolan B, O'Donnell O, Propper C, Puffer F, Schellhorn M, Sundberg G, Winkelhake O.

Equity in the delivery of health care in Europe and the US. *J Health Econ* 2000;**19**:553-83.

9. van Doorslaer E, Masseria C, the OECD Health Equity Research Group Members. Income-Related Inequality in the Use of Medical Care in 21 OECD Countries. 14. 2004. Paris, OECD. OECD Health working papers.

10. Koolman X, van Doorslaer E. On the interpretation of a concentration index of inequality. *Health Econ* 2004;**13**:649-56.

11. The Danish Medicines Agency. Lægemiddelstatistik 1997-2001 [Medicinal Product Statistics 1997-2001]. 2002. Schultz Information.

12. Ministry of Interior and Health. Sundhedssektoren i tal [The Health Care Sector in Numbers]. 2002. Statens Information.

13. Christiansen T, Enemark U, Clausen J, Poulsen P. Health care and cost containment in Denmark. In: Mossialos E, Le Grand J, editors. Health Care and Cost Containment in the European Union. Ashgate, 1999:267.

14. Henricson K, Stenberg P, Rametsteiner G, Ranstam J, Hanson BS, Melander A. Socioeconomic factors, morbidity and drug utilization - An ecological study. *Pharmacoepidemiol Drug Safe* 1998;**7**:261-67.

15. Metge C, Black C, Peterson S, Kozyrskyj AL. The population's use of pharmaceuticals. *Med Care* 1999;**37**:JS42-JS59.

16. Lexchin J. Income class and pharmaceutical expenditure in Canada: 1964-1990. *Can J Public Health* 1996;**87**:46-50.

17. Eggen AE. Pattern of drug use in a general population--prevalence and predicting factors: the Tromso study. *Int J Epidemiol* 1994;**23**:1262-72.

18. Furu K, Straume B, Thelle DS. Legal drug use in a general population: association with gender, morbidity, health care utilization, and lifestyle characteristics. *J Clin Epidemiol* 1997;**50**:341-49.

19. van der Meer JB, van den Bos J, Mackenbach JP. Socioeconomic differences in the utilization of health services in a Dutch population: the contribution of health status. *Health Policy* 1996;**37**:1-18.

20. Kjøller M, Rasmussen NK. Danish Health and Morbidity Survey 2000 ... & trends since 1989. 2002. National Institute of Public Health.

21. Christiansen T. Equity in the Delivery of Health Care in Denmark. CHS Working Paper. University of Southern Denmark 1997;**10**.

22. Gundgaard J, Sørensen J. Evaluering af Fyns Amts Forebyggelsesstrategi: Baseline survey om sundhedstilstand og adfærd omkring tobak, alcohol, kost og motion [Evaluation of the Prevention Strategy in Funen County: Baseline Survey on Behaviour with respct to Tobacco, Alcohol, Diet and Exercise]. 2002. Funen County.

23. Hallas J, Nissen A. Individualized drug utilization statistics. Analysing a population's drug use from the perspective of individual users. *Eur J Clin Pharmacol* 1994;**47**:367-72.

24. Hallas J. Conducting pharmacoepidemiologic research in Denmark. *Pharmacoepidemiol Drug Safe* 2001;**10**:619-23.

25. Brooks R. EuroQol: the current state of play. *Health Policy* 1996;**37**:53-72.

26. Dolan P. Modeling valuations for EuroQol health states. *Med Care* 1997;**35**:1095-108.

27. The EuroQol Group. EuroQol--a new facility for the measurement of health-related quality of life. *Health Policy* 1990;**16**:199-208.

28. Wittrup-Jensen KU, Lauridsen J, Gudex C, Brooks R, Pedersen KM. Danish EuroQol tariffs estimated by the Visual Analogue Scale (VAS) and the Time Trade-Off (TTO). Paper presented at the 6th EuroQol Group Meeting in Copenhagen, 6/7 September 2001. Not yet published 2001.

29. Lipscomb J, Ancukiewicz M, Parmigiani G, Hasselblad V, Samsa G, Matchar DB. Predicting the cost of illness: a comparison of alternative models applied to stroke. *Med Decis Making* 1998;**18**:S39-S56.

30. Manning WG. The logged dependent variable, heteroscedasticity, and the retransformation problem. *J Health Econ* 1998;**17**:283-95.

31. Andersen CK, Andersen K, Kragh-Sorensen P. Cost function estimation: The choice of a model to apply to dementia. *Health Econ* 2000;**9**:397-409.

32. Mackenbach JP, Kunst AE. Measuring the magnitude of socio-economic inequalities in health: an overview of available measures illustrated with two examples from Europe. *Soc Sci Med* 1997;**44**:757-71.

33. Wagstaff A, Paci P, van Doorslaer E. On the measurement of inequalities in health. *Soc Sci Med* 1991;**33**:545-57.

34. Van der Heyden JH, Demarest S, Tafforeau J, Van Oyen H. Socio-economic differences in the utilisation of health services in Belgium. *Health Policy* 2003;**65**:153-65.

Chapter 3

Income-related inequality in utilization of health services in Denmark: Evidence from Funen County

Jens Gundgaard

Abstract

Aims: To examine income-related inequity in utilization of healthcare services in Denmark.

Methods: A health survey of 2,915 respondents in Funen County interviewed in 2000 and 2001 on health status and socioeconomic and sociodemographic characteristics was merged with various computerized registers including inpatient stays, ambulatory visits, contacts in the primary health care sector, and prescription medicine. The index of horizontal inequity was used to estimate the degree of horizontal inequity in utilization of healthcare services across income groups, using the indirect method of standardization to control for age, gender and self-assessed health as a proxy for need. The standardization method rests on the assumption of equal response behaviour across income groups.

Results: The least advantaged with respect to income consume a bigger share of the health services than the most advantaged with the exception of dental treatments where the opposite is true. After standardization for age, gender, and health status there is no significant inequity in use of all healthcare services. However, when it comes to specific healthcare services the least advantaged have a significantly lower share of the medicine consumption and dental treatments than expected.

Conclusion: The index of horizontal inequity suggests that the Danish healthcare system is in general equitable. In sectors with high degree of co-payment some horizontal inequity disfavouring the lower income groups appears to be present.

Key words: Concentration index, healthcare, inequity, social inequality, utilization

Introduction

It is well known that there are social inequalities in health and in use of healthcare.[1-6] Equality in health and equal access to health care are main objectives of health policy in many countries.[7-9] To achieve this goal healthcare in Denmark is mainly financed through general taxation, and universal coverage exists such that financial barriers are minimized. However, for some types of healthcare a considerable degree of co-payment is present. This is the case for dentistry, physiotherapy, and medicine. For dentistry the size of the co-payment is attributable to the specific service and varies between 35% and 100%. For physiotherapy the co-payment is the same percentage for all the services, 61%, although some patients are exempt from co-payment, whereas for prescription medicine the co-payment follows the individual at a decreasing rate, such that large-scale consumers of medicine face a lower percentage of co-payment. For the first DKr 500 of prescription medicine per year the co-payment constitutes 100% of the price.

If utilization of healthcare varies with socioeconomic position even after controlling for socio-demographic characteristics like age and gender, and health status, the distribution and use of healthcare in the population might not follow the overall goal of equal access for equal need. Thus, it would be considered inequitable if use of health care was systematically related to socioeconomic characteristics like income rather than need. Social inequalities in health care can be caused by the financial barriers to access to healthcare services.

The concentration index has become a standard method for measuring income-related inequalities in health and healthcare utilization.[10-14] In van Doorslaer et al. [15] concentration indices have been used on survey data to measure income-related inequalities in hospital utilization, physician, medical specialist, and dental visits as an international comparison between 21 countries. They find that in almost all countries the least advantaged with respect to income have more visits to the general practitioner than the most advantaged. After controlling for the fact that need for healthcare is also concentrated more among the least advantaged, inequalities favouring the better off are found in about half the countries. In most countries, including Denmark, the higher income groups see a specialist more frequently after controlling for need, and in all countries the higher income groups go to the dentist more often. No clear pattern emerges for inpatient hospitalization.

Utilization analyses have also been carried out in more traditional fashion with traditional regression analysis instead of concentration indices. A Belgian study about socioeconomic differences in the utilization of health services found that people with low socioeconomic status more often use GP services, nursing care at home, and are more often admitted to hospitals. However, after adjustment for health status, people with high socioeconomic status report more frequent consumption of specialist, physiotherapist, and dental services.[16]

A similar Dutch study showed higher utilization rates of healthcare for lower educational groups compared with those who have an academic background. Controlling for sociodemographic background variables and health status, the differences diminished (GP services) or reversed (specialist services) the relationship across educational groups.[5]

In most utilization studies utilization of healthcare services has been proxied by the number of contacts or the imputed value of reported number of contacts from health surveys.[5,14,16] The purpose of the present study is to measure the extent of socioeconomic inequalities in utilization of healthcare services in Denmark in monetary terms using data from computerized registers and a health survey.

Material and methods

Subjects

The data set used for the analysis is a combination of survey data and individual level administrative databases. A total of 5,000 people living in Funen County, Denmark aged 16-80 were drawn from The Centralised Civil Register to participate in a health survey on health status, health behaviour, and socioeconomic background. The sample was stratified with regard to municipalities, and the respondents have been weighted by the reciprocals of their selection probabilities (not taking internal non-response into account). The data were gathered through telephone interviews that took place in the period from October 2000 to April 2001.

The survey data were merged with data from individual-level computerized registers including all somatic hospital visits, visits in the primary healthcare sector and prescription medicine in 2000 and 2001. Healthcare services were measured as the costs of the services and approximated by prices, charges, or fees.

The hospital visits were extracted from Funen County Patient Administrative Database (FPAS), which includes records on all inpatient stays, plus ambulatory and emergency room visits. Each hospital admission was described by an estimated charge based on the 2002 Danish case mix system of Diagnosis Related Groups (DRGs). The case-mix system covers inpatient hospital stays, whereas ambulatory and emergency room visits are described by a similar but a more simple system. Capital costs are not included in the case-mix system. All charges were adjusted to 2003 price level for hospital treatments.

The visits in the primary healthcare sector were extracted from the Registry of Public Health Insurance. This registry includes all partly or fully reimbursed health services in the primary healthcare sector, i.e. from general practitioners, physiotherapists, dentists, and specialists. Each service is described with a reimbursement fee. As considerable co-payment exists for healthcare services from the dentist and the physiotherapist these fees have been adjusted to calculate the total amounts (reimbursement + co-payment). Expert judgements were used to adjust the dentist fees to the average level of Funen dentist fees, whereas the relevant physiotherapist fees where adjusted by dividing the reimbursement fees with the proportion of reimbursement. All reimbursement fees were inflation adjusted to 2003 by the price index for physician and physiotherapist services. General practitioners are partly financed through capitation (about one third of GP income). The capitation has not been allocated to the different services as this would have been rather arbitrary, and is therefore excluded from the analysis.

Medicine was determined from the Odense University Pharmacoepidemiologic Database (OPED). This database consists of all prescription refunds from Funen County. Each purchase of reimbursed medicine from a pharmacy in Funen County is described by a pharmacy retail price including value-added tax. Medicine used at hospitals is included in the hospital charges. Furthermore, the database does not contain information on over-the-counter-medicine and prescription medicine not entitled to reimbursement.[17] The pharmacy retail prices were inflation adjusted to 2003 level by the index for pharmaceutical products and equipment.

Variables

Table I includes a list of variables used in the study. Healthcare utilization is measured in monetary terms (DKr) according to the relevant fees and charges for the services used. There are variables for each type of care, and an aggregate variable with all the types of care together.

Income is measured by gross income the previous year taken from the health survey. Income is a categorical variable consisting of 17 intervals. The sample population is ranked according to the categories. Within each category the respondents are ordered randomly. The ranking of income is used to calculate the fractional income rank according to Lerman et al. where the weighting of the respondents is taken into account.[18]

Gender is measured by a dummy variable for being female and age is a continuous variable. Health status is included as a proxy for need. Two variables are used. One variable consists of values from the generic health instrument EQ-5D.[19] These values are represented at an interval scale from 1 (perfect health) to 0 (death). Negative values are allowed for health states worse than death. Danish *Time Trade Off* weights were used to calculate the values.[20] The other measure is a dummy vector with categorical answers to a question about general health. The categories can be seen in Table I.

Additional control variables in the study include dummy vectors for education, occupational and marital status, and lifestyle. Lifestyle is measured by dummy variables for being a daily smoker, having a high weekly intake of alcohol (more than 21/14 units of alcohol for men/women), a daily intake of fruits and vegetables, and a sedentary lifestyle.

Table I. Variable list[1]

Variable group	Variable Name	Explanation
Dependent variables	HOSPITAL	Hospital costs for inpatient stays, ambulatory visits, and emergency rooms, DRG-charges and ambulatory charges, DKK.
	GP	Sum of general physician fees, DKK.
	SPECIALIST	Sum of specialist fees, DKK.
	PHYSIO	Sum of physiotherapist fees, DKK.
	DENTIST	Sum of dentist fees, DKK.
	MEDICINE	Prescription medicine (pharmacies' retail prices), DKK.
	AGGREGATE	Aggregated health care costs (sum of all fees and charges), DKK.
SES	INCOME	Gross income the previous year, DKK.
Age and gender	FEMALE	Dummy variable: Female=1, Male=0.
	AGE	Age.
	AGE2	Age to the power of 2.
	AGE3	Age to the power of 3.
Need proxies	EQVALUE	EQ-5D value, Danish TTO weights.
	EXCELLENT	General health: Excellent.
	VERYGOOD	General health: Very good.
	GOOD	General health: Good.
	FAIR	General health: Fair.
	POOR	General health: Poor.

[1] All variables are measured at individual level

Working sample

In total, 5,000 people from Funen County were drawn from The Centralised Civil Register to participate in the study. However, due to non-response not all participated. 1,578 people were not interviewed for the health survey as they refused to participate, were not found, or were not able to participate for some other reason. This resulted in a survey of 3,422 respondents and an external response rate of 68%. However, not all the respondents answered all the relevant questions and had to be excluded from the study. The final working sample is thus 2,915 respondents with a response rate of 58%.

A descriptive response/non-response analysis has been carried out to shed some light on the differences between the participants and the non-participants. Table II shows means and period prevalence proportions for the relevant variables for the two-year period. There is about the same number of women as men in the working sample. The participants are on average slightly younger than the non-participants. Table II also shows that almost everyone has consumed healthcare services over the two-year course. As could be expected the non-respondents use more healthcare than the respondents (although the proportion of users is not higher). This is the case for almost all the types of healthcare with the exception of physiotherapy and dentistry where the consumption of services is higher for the respondents than the non-respondents.

Table II. Descriptive statistics for respondents and non-respondents[1]

	Participants (2915)		Non-participants (2085)	
	Mean	(Prev. of consumers)	Mean	(Prev. of consumers)
Woman	0.49		0.52	
Age	44.65		46.60	
Hospital costs, DKK	11686	(0.43)	16241	(0.48)
GP costs, DKK	1235	(0.93)	1429	(0.91)
Physiotherapy, DKK	369	(0.10)	320	(0.09)
Specialist, DKK	546	(0.36)	558	(0.35)
Dentist, DKK	1639	(0.78)	1430	(0.69)
Prescription medicin, DKK	2335	(0.76)	3285	(0.78)
Aggregated costs, DKK	17810	(0.98)	23263	(0.97)

Notes: Data not weighted

Statistical analyses

The paper follows the methods described in van Doorslaer et al. [14] and Kakwani et al. [12]. The degree of income-related inequality in consumption of healthcare services is quantified by the index of horizontal inequity, HI_{WV} (where WV is referring to the originators of the index [14]), which is based on concentration indices, and includes standardization for relevant need-based variables. A concentration curve for healthcare consumption is the cumulative proportion of healthcare as a function of the cumulative proportion of the population ranked by socioeconomic status (in this case income).

There are several methods of quantifying inequalities.[21,22] Compared to other indices the HI_{WV} index has some advantages that are worth mentioning: (i) the inequalities in health care consumption are analyzed with respect to socioeconomic status; (ii) the measure includes the whole sampled population, not just the lower and upper income groups; (iii) the index is sensitive to changes in the distribution of the population across income groups; (iv) the index can be illustrated graphically (as in Figure 1); (v) the index can be tested for statistical significance by using regression analysis to estimate the index coefficients.[13]

Fig. I. Example of concentration curves

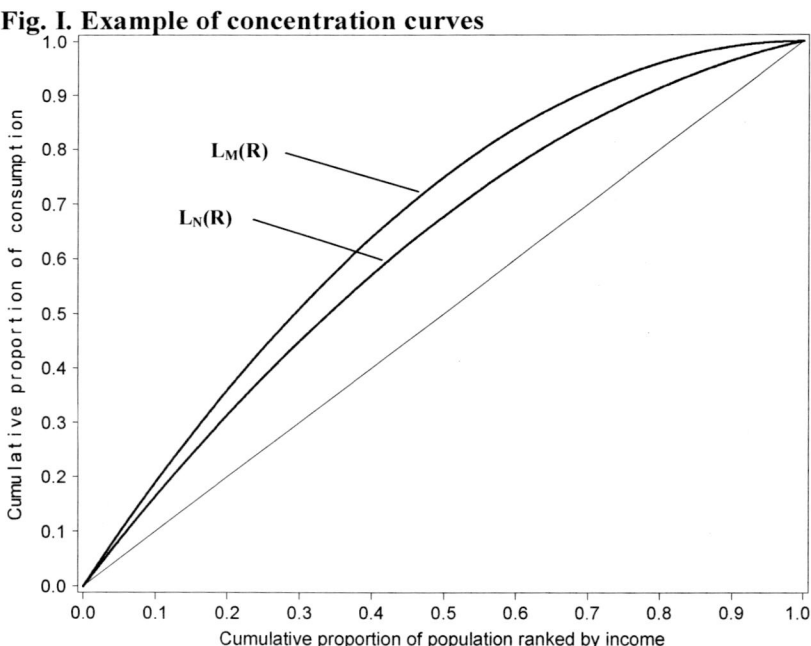

Notes: $L_m(R)$ = Observed concentration curve, $L_n(R)$ = Concentration curve for need.

The concentration curve is illustrated in Figure 1 and denoted $L_M(R)$, where M stands for medical treatment and R is the relative rank. The concentration curve is expected to be concave towards the origin, as the disadvantaged groups with regard to income tend to have a relatively higher consumption of healthcare. The concentration index C is then twice the area between $L_M(R)$ and the 45-degree line in Figure 1 and ranges between 1 and -1. If the concentration curve is concave C will be negative, indicating inequality in favour of the lower income groups and vice versa for convex concentration curves. The concentration index is only an appropriate measure for horizontal inequity as long as individuals are expected to have the same level of consumption, that is, a distribution that follows the 45-degree line in Figure 1. However, older people and people with health problems are expected to be in higher need of healthcare, and a higher level of healthcare among those groups will seldom be characterized as inequitable. Consequently, distribution of actual consumption should be compared to what could be expected due to variation in need (predicted consumption) as opposed to an equal distribution. The quantification of inequality can be standardized indirectly by predicting the expected level of consumption for the individual given age, gender and health status, which works as a proxy for need, and comparing it to actual need. That way the properties of the index are maintained. By using the indirect standardization method it is assumed that individuals at a given income level will have the same consumption as the rest of the population when adjusting for age, gender, and health status. As is normal for healthcare data, consumption of healthcare is badly skewed to the right.[23,24] That is, a few people have a high level of consumption whereas most people have a low level of consumption. A considerable fraction of the population does not have any consumption at all, which exacerbates the skewness and complicates the estimation procedures. To tackle the problem generated by the zero-consumption observations, a two-part regression model is used to predict the level of healthcare consumption for each individual. The two-part model consists of a logistic regression model to predict the probability of having non-zero consumption (part 1), and a semi-log linear regression model to predict the level of consumption given non-zero consumption (part 2). The dependent variable is log transformed to remove the skewness of the distribution.[23] Including only age, gender and health status in the model can lead to omitted variable bias. Therefore, to follow the lines of van Doorslaer et al. [25] additional variables such as income, education, occupational status, marital status, lifestyle variables are added to the model. Their effect is neutralized by setting the values equal to the means when predicting healthcare consumption. However, due to the non-linearity of the two-part model, the effect is not completely neutralized.

The advantage of using a two-part model is that the probability of using healthcare services and the level of health services consumed for consumers are described by different functions as it is probably not the same mechanisms that determine the barriers of starting to consume as the amount of healthcare consumed for people who are already consumers.

A concentration curve for predicted consumption $L_N(R)$ is also illustrated in Figure 1 (N for need). For calculating the index of horizontal inequity the concentration curve $L_M(R)$ is compared with $L_N(R)$ as opposed to the 45-degree line. Approximate standard errors and t-statistics to calculate 95% confidence intervals are obtained from regression analyses. The index coefficients can be estimated by regressing the relative consumption multiplied by twice the variance of the fractional income rank on the fractional income rank. The OLS estimator for the coefficient of the fractional income rank is equivalent to the HI_{WV} index.[14]

Results

The coefficients from the two-part model used for the standardization procedure are presented in Table III. The two parts of the model include the same explanatory variables, that is, a dummy for gender, a polynomial function of age, and an EQ-5D value. The first part of the two-part model indicates that women have a significantly higher probability of being consumers of healthcare for most types of healthcare, except for hospital visits, and among people who are already consumers women tend to have a higher level of consumption for some types of healthcare (the second part). Age taken to the power of two or three is included in the two-part specifications when the coefficients are significant. The probability of being consumers and the level of consumption increase with age, and is fitted well by polynomial regression in most cases. The EQ-5D variable is a proxy for need and the coefficient for the EQ-5D variable is negative in the two parts. That is, a higher health status diminishes consumption of healthcare. Using a two-part model to solve the zero consumption problem and a semilog model to diminish the skewness makes the residuals approximately normally distributed. The two-part models have been repeated with the general health dummy vector in lieu of the EQ-5D variable. The change in variables for health status does not have any substantial impact on the models' conclusions and the results are left out for the sake of brevity.

The concentration indices and the HI_{WV} indices are given in Table IV. The observed concentration indices are all negative with the exception of dentistry (although not significantly for specialist services and physiotherapy). This means that for most types of care the least advantaged with regard to income consume a bigger share of the health services than the most advantaged. For dentistry the observed concentration index is positive, which means that the concentration curve is convex toward the origin and the most advantaged consume a bigger share of the services.

After standardization for age, gender and health status there is no significant inequity in use of all healthcare services or for most types of healthcare services. However, the least advantaged have a significantly lower share of the medicine consumption and dental treatments than expected. The HI_{WV} index for physiotherapy treatments is also large and positive, although not statistically significant. For GP visits, on the other hand, the HI_{WV} is positive and significant when using the self-assessed health variable as a need proxy. However, the index value is small.

Discussion

For this study a health survey was merged with various individual level computerized registers to analyze income-related inequality in healthcare in Denmark. The analysis shows that the least advantaged with regard to income consume a bigger share of the services than the most advantaged. This is in accordance with previous studies.[5,15,26,27] After indirect standardization for age, gender, and health status there is no significant horizontal inequity. This suggests that the Danish healthcare system is in general equitable. In sectors with high degrees of co-payment a different picture emerges. For specific types of care the least advantaged have a lower share of the medicine consumption and dentistry than expected. For physiotherapy this is also the case, although the index is not statistically significant. This suggests that co-payment has an influence on the level of consumption, and some horizontal inequity favouring the better off is present for these types of care. For GP visits there is also horizontal inequity when using the self-assessed health variable as a need proxy (but not for the EQ-5D variable). However, the magnitude is small and barely significant.

Using registers to extract information on healthcare utilization made it possible to obtain exact information about the healthcare services for a long period. The registers also made it possible to distinguish between types of healthcare that have normally not been included in previous studies: physiotherapy and prescription medicine. The healthcare services have been measured in monetary terms. The advantage of using a common unit of measurement is that different types of services can be added together. Furthermore, the different services are weighted by the importance: a visit is not just a visit. Check-ups, for example, are weighted less than surgical treatments. Nevertheless, the charges and fees used are only crude approximations.

The survey data made it possible to gather information on variables such as self-perceived health status that can normally not be found in registers. The use of survey data, however, limited the size of the sample, which could have been considerably bigger, had the data set only consisted of registers.

The use of survey data also caused non-response. The non-response analysis suggested that the non-respondents had a higher level of healthcare consumption than respondents. The survey data were gathered through telephone interviews. This means that people too weak to have a telephone conversation obviously are not included in the study. This could be one explanation for the higher level of healthcare consumption among the non-respondents for most types of healthcare.

The income variable was taken from the health survey. Income is a sensitive question and a large fraction of the respondents were reluctant to answer that question. Altogether, 485 respondents were left out of the

Table III. Two part model for healthcare costs: Coefficients for the relations between healthcare consumption and explanatory variables

Part 1: Logistic regression[1]

Variable	Hospital	GP	Specialist	Physio.	Dentist	Medicine	Aggregate
INTERCEPT	3.9200 **	9.0188 **	-0.2476	-3.0513	-4.0642 **	2.9396 *	13.9306 **
FEMALE	0.0627	1.3369 **	0.4680 **	0.5236 **	0.3731 **	0.7604 **	0.7573
AGE	-0.1029 **	-0.1274 **	-0.0665 **	0.0052	0.1273 **	-0.0676 *	-0.1819 *
AGE2	0.0010 **	0.0013 *	0.0008 **		-0.0014 **	0.0008 **	0.0018 *
EQVALUE	-2.8230 **	-4.5529 **	-1.8087 **	-3.1911 **	-0.3861	-3.1540 **	-6.1781 **
Observations[3]	2915	2915	2915	2915	2915	2915	2915
Positive consumption	1258.9	2712.6	1061.4	315.8	2315.3	2173.3	2865.4
Zero consumption	1656.1	202.4	1853.6	2599.2	599.7	741.7	49.6
Likelihood Ratio test:							
χ^2	217.94	161.92	219.10	175.67	310.34	274.49	73.25
P-value	<0.0001	<0.0001	<0.0001	<0.0001	<0.0001	<0.0001	<0.0001

Table III. (Continued)

Part 2: Semilog regression[2]

Variable	Hospital		GP		Specialist		Physio.		Dentist		Medicine		Aggregate	
INTERCEPT	9.4480	**	7.7761	**	6.5864	**	6.2342	**	5.5301	**	7.0454	**	9.5668	**
FEMALE	-0.0557		0.4558	**	0.0754		0.0811		0.0115		0.2575	**	0.3029	**
AGE	-0.0459	*	0.0145		0.0041		0.0018		0.0118	**	0.0450	**	-0.0316	*
AGE2	0.0005	*	-0.0010										0.0005	**
AGE3			0.0000	*										
EQVALUE	-1.6882	**	-1.7456	**	-0.6283	**	-1.5602	**	-0.2846	**	-2.0969	**	-2.6382	**
Observations[3]	1258.9		2712.6		1061.4		315.8		2315.3		2173.3		2865.4	
F-value	8.4218		18.2801		1.4768		2.7334		10.9608		29.8464		28.2397	
P-value	<0.0001		<0.0001		0.0532		<0.0001		<0.0001		<0.0001		<0.0001	
R^2	0.1719		0.1747		0.0391		0.2165		0.1234		0.2835		0.2304	

Notes: [1]Part 1: Logistic regression for the probability of healthcare consumption. [2]Part 2: Level of healthcare consumption given non-zero consumption. Coefficients for 27 control variables (log of income, education, occupational status, marital status, lifestyle variables) are not shown. [3]Data weighted by the reciprocals of the sampling probability and normalized to the sample size. Statistical significance assessed using Wald χ^2 and t-test as appropriate. Tests based on stratification adjusted standard errors. *p<0.05, **p<0.01

Tabel IV. Concentration indices and HI indices for healthcare consumption over a two-year period[1]

	Need proxy	C_M	95% CI[2] 95L	95% CI[2] 95U	C_N	95% CI[2] 95L	95% CI[2] 95U	HI	95% CI[2] 95L	95% CI[2] 95U
Hospital	EQ-5D TTO-value	-0.1908	-0.2970	-0.0846	-0.1460	-0.1641	-0.1279	-0.0448	-0.1481	0.0585
	Health variable	-0.1908	-0.2970	-0.0846	-0.1715	-0.1907	-0.1522	-0.0193	-0.1218	0.0832
GP	EQ-5D TTO-value	-0.1051	-0.1298	-0.0803	-0.1231	-0.1367	-0.1096	0.0180	-0.0045	0.0406
	Health variable	-0.1051	-0.1298	-0.0803	-0.1279	-0.1402	-0.1157	0.0228	0.0008	0.0449
Specialist	EQ-5D TTO-value	-0.0479	-0.1279	0.0322	-0.0970	-0.1079	-0.0861	0.0492	-0.0298	0.1282
	Health variable	-0.0479	-0.1279	0.0322	-0.1081	-0.1197	-0.0965	0.0602	-0.0185	0.1390
Physiotherapist	EQ-5D TTO-value	-0.0520	-0.1522	0.0482	-0.1463	-0.1858	-0.1068	0.0943	-0.0038	0.1924
	Health variable	-0.0520	-0.1522	0.0482	-0.1295	-0.1576	-0.1014	0.0775	-0.0198	0.1748
Dentist	EQ-5D TTO-value	0.1019	0.0810	0.1227	0.0136	0.0082	0.0189	0.0883	0.0681	0.1086
	Health variable	0.1019	0.0810	0.1227	0.0182	0.0132	0.0232	0.0837	0.0634	0.1039
Prescription medicine	EQ-5D TTO-value	-0.0920	-0.1427	-0.0412	-0.1702	-0.2067	-0.1338	0.0782	0.0293	0.1272
	Health variable	-0.0920	-0.1427	-0.0412	-0.1860	-0.2197	-0.1522	0.0940	0.0461	0.1419
Aggregated costs	EQ-5D TTO-value	-0.1364	-0.2079	-0.0649	-0.1267	-0.1539	-0.0995	-0.0097	-0.0807	0.0613
	Health variable	-0.1364	-0.2079	-0.0649	-0.1311	-0.1530	-0.1092	-0.0053	-0.0736	0.0630

Notes: [1]The HI_{WV}-index is indirectly standardized by two-part models including age, gender and a health status measure: EQ-5D TTO-value or a self-assessed health variable. Data weighted by the reciprocals of the sampling probability and normalized to the sample size. [2]95% confidence intervals based on stratification adjusted standard errors analysis due to missing observations with regard to income. Furthermore, the answers could be subject to recall bias, as not all people might remember their exact gross income from the previous year. On the other hand, the answers are given in income categories and the concentration indices might not be that sensitive to the precision of the income.

The study covers only services that are subject to partial or complete reimbursement by the Public Health Insurance. For most types of healthcare there is no co-payment (although private for-profit supply of some healthcare services does exist). For dentistry, however, a considerable share of the services is not reimbursed at all, and these services are not included in the database. If income-related inequalities exist they are probably bigger for the kind of services the patients have to pay for. Therefore, the concentration index for dentistry is certainly a conservative estimate.

For medicine, only prescription medicines in the primary healthcare sector entitled to reimbursement are in the database. Prescription medicine bought from pharmacies outside Funen County, medicine used in hospitals, and illegal purchases of medicine over the internet are not covered by the database (medicine used in hospitals is included in hospital charges).

The healthcare data were limited to two years (2000 and 2001). The longer the period, the smaller the problem of zero-consumption data and random fluctuations. However, the health status indicators are point estimates, and will be less valid as standardization variables for healthcare consumption that has occurred too long before or after the time of the interview.

As a proxy for need for healthcare consumption two measures for health status were used: EQ-5D values and general self-assessed health. Health status as a proxy for need for healthcare services is common in the literature.[5,14-16] Self-reported health status is not always a good proxy for need for healthcare. It rests on the assumption that people have the same understanding of health across income groups. It is possible that the lower income groups have a more pessimistic view of their life in general and therefore also of their health status. This will overestimate their need and exaggerate the inequality estimates. The opposite can also be the case if the higher income groups underestimate their good health and/or the lower income groups underestimate their bad health due to adaptation. However, unless we have a more objective measure of need we cannot quantify this reference bias.[25,28,29] Furthermore, some products are taken for the preventive effect. When treatment cures the illnesses the need for healthcare is not accounted for by the health status indicators, which might show good or perfect health as a result of the treatment. For dental care the health status variables seem to be particularly inappropriate as general health status cannot be expected to be a good proxy for dental health status. In addition, the standardization implies that the consumption is assumed to be right on average given the explanatory variables. If this is not the case, or if the econometric specifications are not unbiased, then the standardization can do more harm than good. The predicted concentration index for dental treatments is positive. However, a Danish study has shown that dental health status is negatively correlated with socioeconomic status.[30] The HI_{WV} for dentistry is therefore very likely a conservative estimate of horizontal inequity in dental services.

Conclusion

Health survey data were merged with individual level administrative databases to analyze income- related inequality in utilization of healthcare. The analysis shows that the least advantaged with regard to income consume a bigger share of the healthcare than the most advantaged. The healthcare consumption is standardized with an indirect standardization method. The method rests on the assumption of equal response behaviour across income groups. After standardization for age, gender, and health status no significant inequality is present for healthcare services at an aggregate level. However, for types of healthcare with high co-payment rates, dentistry and prescription medicine, inequality favouring the most advantaged is found, and this suggests that for some types of healthcare horizontal inequity favouring the higher income groups is present.

Acknowledgements

The author would like to thank Funen County for delivery of hospital data and OPED for delivery of prescription records. The study was carried out thanks to a research grant from The Health Insurance Foundation, Denmark (Sygekassernes Helsefond). The author alone is responsible for the contents of the article.

References

1. Kunst AE, Mackenbach JP. The size of mortality differences associated with educational level in nine industrialized countries. *Am J Public Health* 1994;**84**:932-37.

2. Mackenbach JP, Kunst AE, Cavelaars AE, Groenhof F, Geurts JJ. Socioeconomic inequalities in morbidity and mortality in western Europe. The EU Working Group on Socioeconomic Inequalities in Health. *Lancet* 1997;**349**:1655-59.

3. Gerdtham UG, Sundberg G. Equity in the delivery of health care in Sweden. *Scand J Soc Med* 1998;**26**:259-64.

4. Merlo J, Gerdtham UG, Lynch J, Beckman A, Norlund A, Lithman T. Social inequalities in health- do they diminish with age? Revisiting the question in Sweden 1999. *Int J Equity Health* 2003;**2**:2.

5. van der Meer JB, van den Bos J, Mackenbach JP. Socioeconomic differences in the utilization of health services in a Dutch population: the contribution of health status. *Health Policy* 1996;**37**:1-18.

6. Avlund K, Holstein BE, Osler M, Damsgaard MT, Holm-Pedersen P, Rasmussen NK. Social position and health in old age: the relevance of different indicators of social position. *Scand J Public Health* 2003;**31**:126-36.

7. Dahlgren G, Whitehead M. Policies and strategies to promote equity in health. 1-50. 2000. Copenhagen, WHO Regional Office for Europe.

8. The Copenhagen declaration on reducing social inequalities in health. *Scand J Public Health* 2002;**Suppl 59**:78-79.

9. Stronks G, Gunning-Schepers LJ. Should equity in health be target number 1. *Eur J Public Health* 1993;**65**:153-65.

10. Clarke PM, Gerdtham UG, Connelly LB. A note on the decomposition of the health concentration index. *Health Econ* 2003;**12**:511-16.

11. Humphries KH, van Doorslaer E. Income-related health inequality in Canada. *Soc Sci Med* 2000;**50**:663-71.

12. Kakwani N, Wagstaff A, van Doorslaer E. Socioeconomic Inequalities in Health: Measurement, Computation, and Statistical Inference. *J Econometrics* 1997;**77**:87-103.

13. van Doorslaer E, Wagstaff A, Bleichrodt H, Calonge S, Gerdtham UG, Gerfin, M, Geurts J, Gross L, Häkkinen U, Leu RE, O'Donnell O, Propper C, Puffer F, Rodríguez M, Sundberg G, Winkelhake O. Income-related inequalities in health: some international comparisons. *J Health Econ* 1997;**16**:93-112.

14. van Doorslaer E, Wagstaff A, van der Burg H, Christiansen T, De Graeve D, Duchesne I, Gerdtham UG, Gerfin M, Geurts J, Gross L, Häkkinen U, John J, Klavus J, Leu RE, Nolan B, O'Donnell O, Propper C, Puffer F, Schellhorn M, Sundberg G, Winkelhake O. Equity in the delivery of health care in Europe and the US. *J Health Econ* 2000;**19**:553-83.

15. van Doorslaer E, Masseria C, the OECD Health Equity Research Group Members. Income-Related Inequality in the Use of Medical Care in 21 OECD Countries. 14. 2004. Paris, OECD. OECD Health working papers.

16. Van der Heyden JH, Demarest S, Tafforeau J, Van Oyen H. Socio-economic differences in the utilisation of health services in Belgium. *Health Policy* 2003;**65**:153-65.

17. Hallas J. Conducting pharmacoepidemiologic research in Denmark. *Pharmacoepidemiol Drug Safe* 2001;**10**:619-23.

18. Lerman RI, Yitzhaki S. Improving the Accuracy of Estimates of Gini-Coefficients. *J Econometrics* 1989;**42**:43-47.

19. Brooks R. EuroQol: the current state of play. *Health Policy* 1996;**37**:53-72.

20. Wittrup-Jensen KU, Lauridsen J, Gudex C, Brooks R, Pedersen KM. Estimating Danish EQ-5D tariffs using the Time Trade-Off (TTO) and visual analogue scale (VAS) methods. In: Norinder AL, Pedersen KM, Roos P (editors). Proceedings of the 18th Plenary Meeting of the EuroQol Group. 6-7 September 2001, Copenhagen, Denmark, IHE – The Swedish Institute for Health Economics, Lund.

21. Wagstaff A, Paci P, van Doorslaer E. On the measurement of inequalities in health. *Soc Sci Med* 1991;**33**:545-57.

22. Mackenbach JP, Kunst AE. Measuring the magnitude of socio-economic inequalities in health: an overview of available measures illustrated with two examples from Europe. *Soc Sci Med* 1997;**44**:757-71.

23. Manning WG. The logged dependent variable, heteroscedasticity, and the retransformation problem. *J Health Econ* 1998;**17**:283-95.

24. Lipscomb J, Ancukiewicz M, Parmigiani G, Hasselblad V, Samsa G, Matchar DB. Predicting the cost of illness: a comparison of

alternative models applied to stroke. *Med Decis Making* 1998;**18**:S39-S56.

25. van Doorslaer E, Koolman X, Jones AM. Explaining income-related inequalities in doctor utilisation in Europe. *Health Econ* 2004;**13**:629-47.

26. Metge C, Black C, Peterson S, Kozyrskyj AL. The population's use of pharmaceuticals. *Med Care* 1999;**37**:JS42-JS59.

27. Lexchin J. Income class and pharmaceutical expenditure in Canada: 1964-1990. *Can J Public Health* 1996;**87**:46-50.

28. Groot W. Adaptation and scale of reference bias in self-assessments of quality of life
2. *J Health Econ* 2000;**19**:403-20.

29. Jürges H. Self-assessed health, reference points, and mortality. MEA Discussion Paper 57-04 2005.

30. Petersen PE, Kjøller M, Christensen LB. Adult dental health status and use of oral healht services in Denmark 2000. Sociobehavioural determinants for improvement in oral health [in Danish]. *Tandlaegebladet.* 2003;**107**:672-84.

Chapter 4

Explaining the Sources of Income-Related Inequality in Health Care Utilization in Denmark

Jens Gundgaard, Jørgen Lauridsen

Submitted to
International Journal of Health Care Finance and Economics

Abstract

Objectives with the health care system often include equity considerations. One objective is equal treatment for equal need. In this paper we explain the sources of income-related inequality in utilization of health care services in Funen County, Denmark, by linking survey data to register based data. A decomposition of the concentration index was used to explain the sources of overall income-related inequality in utilization. The decomposition approach suggests that health care is in general equally distributed in Denmark when need based variables are controlled for. However, this overall result is a consequence of a number of off-setting effects from different types of health care and a complicated pattern of various explanatory variables.

Key words: health care, utilization, concentration index, inequality, decomposition

Introduction

The concentration index has become the standard method of estimating the degree of income-related inequality in utilization of health care.[1,2] It is well known that there are inequalities in use of some types of health care. Lately, there has also been an increased focus on the sources of this inequality.[3,4] In several studies decompositions of concentration indices have been used to investigate the contributions to the magnitude of the inequality.[3-7] Furthermore, the decomposition approach can also be used to directly standardize for need.[8] The principle for most studies of health care utilization is that people in equal need should be treated equally.[2,9] Therefore, need has to be taken into account when calculating concentration indices for equitable distributions. Excluding the contributions from need-based variables is equivalent to directly standardizing the concentration index for need[41].[8]

The present paper follows the lines of Clarke et al. [7] and Wagstaff et al. [6] and applied in Lauridsen et al. [10] In Wagstaff et al. a multivariate regression approach was used for a decomposition of background characteristics. The regression approach assisted a decomposition of the single characteristic's impact on income-related inequality in a health into 1) its regressive impact on the variation in health, and 2) the impact due to income-related inequality in the characteristic itself. In Clarke et al. a concentration index of health inequality was decomposed separately by health dimension and subgroup. The decomposition by dimension was a weighted average of concentration indices for each dimension (with the relative share of the aggregate health as weights). In Lauridsen et al. the decomposition by dimension from Clarke et al. was merged with the regression approach from Wagstaff et al. The concentration index was decomposed into the different dimensions of health summing up the index and the effect on health from different socio-economic characteristics.

In the present study the decomposition approach from Lauridsen et al. was applied on health care services.[10] The concentration index for income-related inequality in health care utilization was decomposed into contributions from six different types

---

[41] In the literature the terms 'direct' and 'indirect' standardization are used in different ways. Here the approach from Gravelle is used.

of health care and from various explanatory variables including age, gender, health status, income, education, occupation, marital status and life style variables. The paper adds to existing literature by measuring health care utilization in monetary terms by using register-based data, and by including types of health care and explanatory variables that have not been included in previous studies.

Data

The data set used for the analysis is a combination of survey data and registers. 5,000 people living in Funen County, Denmark aged 16-80 were drawn from The Centralised Civil Register to participate in a health survey on health status, health behavior and socio-economic background. The sample was stratified with respect to municipalities, and the respondents have been weighted by the reciprocals of their selection probabilities (not taking internal non-response into account). The data were gathered through telephone interviews that took place in the period from October 2000 through April 2001.[11]

The survey data were merged with data from individual level computerized registers including all somatic hospital visits, visits in the primary health care sector and prescription medicine in 2000 and 2001. Health care services were measured as the costs of the services and approximated by prices, charges or fees. Using registers to extract information on health care utilization makes it possible to obtain exact information about the health care services for a long period. The registers also make it possible to distinguish between types of health care that have normally not been included in previous studies: physiotherapy and prescription medicine. The health care services have been measured in monetary terms. The advantage of using a common unit of measurement is different types of services can be added together. Furthermore, the different services are weighted by the importance: A visit is not just a visit. Check-ups, for example, are weighted less than surgical treatments. Nevertheless, the charges and fees used are only crude approximations of the quality.

The hospital visits were extracted from Funen County Patient Administrative Database (FPAS), which includes records on all inpatient stays, ambulatory and emergency room visits. Each hospital admission was described by an estimated charge based on the 2002

Danish case mix system of Diagnosis Related Groups (DRGs). The case mix system covers inpatient hospital stays, whereas ambulatory and emergency room visits are described by a similar, but a more simple system. Overhead costs are not included in the case mix system. All charges were adjusted to 2003 price level for hospital treatments.

The visits in the primary health care sector were extracted from The Registry of Public Health Insurance. This registry includes all partly or fully reimbursed health services in the primary health care sector, i.e. from the general practitioners, physiotherapists, dentists and specialists. Each service is described with a reimbursement fee. As considerable co-payment exists for health care services from the dentist and the physiotherapist these fees have been adjusted to get the total amounts (reimbursement + co-payment)[42]. Expert judgments were used to adjust the dentist fees to the average level of Funen dentist fees[43], whereas the relevant physiotherapist fees where adjusted by dividing the reimbursement fees with the proportion of reimbursement[44]. General practitioners are partly financed through capitation (about one third of GP income), and the GP reimbursement fees were scaled up by this amount. All reimbursement fees were inflation adjusted to 2003 by the price index for physicians and physiotherapists. Medicine was from Odense University Pharmacoepidemiologic Database (OPED). This database consists of all prescription refunds from Funen County. Each purchase of reimbursed medicine from a pharmacy in Funen County is described by a pharmacy retail price including VAT[45]. Medicine used at hospitals is included in the hospital charges. Furthermore, the database does not contain information on over-the-counter-medicine and

---

[42] About 18% of all health care expenditures in Denmark are financed directly by the patients.
[43] For dentistry the size of the co-payment is attributable to the specific service and varies between 35% and 100%. Expert judgments were used to get a more accurate description of the price level of the different services as there is no clear relationship between the reimbursements and the full prices.
[44] For physiotherapy the co-payment is the same percentage for all the services, 61%, although some patients are exempt from co-payment.
[45] For prescription medicine the co-payment follows the individual at a decreasing rate, such that large-scale consumers of medicine face a lower percentage of co-payment.

prescription medicine not entitled to reimbursement[46].[12]. The pharmacy retail prices were inflation adjusted to 2003 level by the index for pharmaceutical products and equipment.

The ranking variable for the concentration index was income and this variable was defined as personal gross income from the previous year (gross of tax and deductibles) and measured as a categorical variable with 17 categories. The respondents were ranked according to their income category. Within the categories the respondents were ranked randomly. To follow the practice from the literature the logarithm was taken of income to diminish the skewness for the inclusion of income as an explanatory variable in the regression models[47].[3-5]

Other explanatory variables included age, gender, health status, socio-economic and lifestyle variables. Age and gender were described by categorical age and gender groups. Health status was measured at an interval scale using Danish EQ-5D TTO values. The scale takes values from 1 (perfect health) to 0 (dead). However, some respondents have negative values indicating health states worse than dead[48].[13-16]

Socio-economic variables were represented by dummy vectors for educational, occupational level and marital status. Lifestyle was characterized by dummy variables of being daily smoker, having a high weekly intake of alcohol (more than 21/14 units of alcohol for men/women), a daily intake of fruits and vegetables, and a sedentary lifestyle.

Due to non-response not all 5,000 people participated. 1,578 people were not interviewed for the health survey as they refused to participate, were not found, or were not able to participate for some other reason. This results in a survey of 3,422 respondents and an external response rate of 68 percent. However, not all the respondents answered all the relevant questions and had to be excluded from the study. As is common, income is a sensitive question that some people

---

[46] Prescription medicine such as oral contraceptives, benzodiazepines, and certain antibiotics is not entitled to reimbursement.

[47] As an explanatory variable, income was treated as a continuous variable by using midpoints.

[48] Only five people had negative scores and they were included in the sample.

abstain from answering. Furthermore, people were also excluded due to lack of response to the questions regarding health. For the socio-economic and socio-demographic determinants missing answers were categorized in residual categories (like "other type of education" or "other type of job") in order to maintain people in the sample. The final working samples then consists of 2,915 respondents. This is equivalent to response rates of 58 percent.

Descriptive response/non-response analysis showed that the working sample is representative with respect to socio-demographic characteristics.[11] However, for almost all the types of health care the respondents use less health care than the non-respondents (although the proportion of users is about the same in the two groups)[49].

Modelling

As shown in Kakwani et al. [17] the concentration index C can be estimated by the convenient OLS regression

$$2\sigma^2 \left(\frac{y_i}{\mu} \right) = \alpha + \beta R_i + \varepsilon_i, \quad (1)$$

where the y_i/μ is the relative consumption of health care services for individual i, R_i is the fractional income rank based on weights (the reciprocals of selection probabilities normalised to the sample size), and σ^2 is the variance of the fractional income rank. Then the OLS coefficient of the relative rank, $\hat{\beta}$, is equivalent to C.

For the purpose of decomposing C by income, need-standardizing variables, socio-economic and life style determinants it is assumed that health care is linked to these K determinants through a regression model:

$$y_i = f \left(\beta_I \ln x_{Ii} + \sum_Z \beta_Z x_{Zi} + \sum_S \beta_S x_{Si} + \sum_L \beta_L x_{Li} \right). \quad (2)$$

If formula 2 is a linear regression model then the concentration index can be decomposed as:

---

[49] Presumably a group of people is missing from the survey due to bad health and is expected to have a higher level of consumption of health care than what we se among the respondents.

$$C = \frac{\beta_I \mu_I}{\mu} C_I + \sum_Z \frac{\beta_Z \mu_Z}{\mu} C_Z + \sum_S \frac{\beta_S \mu_S}{\mu} C_S + \sum_L \frac{\beta_L \mu_L}{\mu} C_L + \frac{1}{\mu} CG_\varepsilon \qquad (3)$$

where μ is the mean of y, and μ_k, β_k and C_k the mean, the regression coefficient and the concentration index of kth determinant, respectively.[6] The decomposition is made up of two components: 1) The predicted concentration index, which is a deterministic component equal to the weighted sum of concentration indices of the K regressors, where the weight of x_k is simply the elasticity of y with respect to x_k. 2) A residual component, which is the generalized concentration index for ε, and reflects the income-related inequalities in health care that cannot be explained by variation in income.

If the link between health care and the K determinants is modelled as a non-linear regression model, which is normal for skewed data and data with a high share of zero-observations, then the relation in formula (3) no longer holds. However, a linear relationship can be approximated by the partial effects from a non-linear model.[4]

When aggregate health care is additively composed of health care from different sectors, which will be the case if health care is measured in monetary terms, then the concentration index for y can also be decomposed as a weighted average:

$$C = \sum_j w_j C_j, \qquad (4)$$

where C is the concentration index for y, C_j is the concentration index for sector j, and w_j is a weight attached to the jth sector and estimated as $w_j = \mu_j/\mu$, with μ_j and μ being the means of y and y_j respectively.[7] Each of the C_js can be decomposed as in formula (3). Substituting formula (3) for each sector into formula (4) gives:

$$\begin{aligned} C &= \sum_j w_j C_j \\ &= \sum_j w_j \left[\frac{\beta_{jI} \mu_I}{\mu_j} C_I + \sum_Z \frac{\beta_{jZ} \mu_Z}{\mu_j} C_Z + \sum_S \frac{\beta_{jS} \mu_S}{\mu_j} C_S + \sum_L \frac{\beta_{jL} \mu_L}{\mu_j} C_L + \frac{1}{\mu} CG_{\varepsilon j} \right] \quad (5) \\ &= \sum_j \frac{\beta_{jI} \mu_I}{\mu} C_I + \sum_{j,Z} \frac{\beta_{jZ} \mu_Z}{\mu} C_Z + \sum_{j,S} \frac{\beta_{jS} \mu_S}{\mu} C_S + \sum_{j,L} \frac{\beta_{jL} \mu_L}{\mu} C_L + \sum_j \frac{1}{\mu} CG_{\varepsilon j} \end{aligned}$$

The betas can be estimated from sector specific regression models for health care utilization.[10] This decomposition contains contributions from six different types of health care and from various explanatory variables including age, gender, health status, income, education, occupation, marital status and life style variables.

The concentration index is standardized for need by estimating the augmented partial concentration index as in Gravelle.[8] This is equivalent to the horizontal inequity index in van Doorslaer et al.[4] Gravelle suggests a direct standardization of the need based variables by excluding their contributions from the decomposition[50].

$$HI = C - \sum_{j,z} \frac{\beta_{jz} \mu_z}{\mu} C_z \qquad (6)$$

It is not obvious whether or not the generalized concentration index should count as a contribution to the concentration index or the standardizing component. According to Gravelle both approaches are consistent estimates of the augmented concentration index. The present paper follows the style of van Doorslaer et al. and includes the generalized concentration index in *HI*.[4]

Estimation

As is normal for health care data, the distribution is highly skewed to the right and have many zero-consumption-observations.[18,19] To deal with the problem of zero-consumption observations, a two-part regression model (TPM) is used to predict the level of health care consumption for each individual. The TPM consists of a logistic regression model to predict the probability of having non-zero consumption (part 1), and a semi-log linear regression model to predict the level of consumption given non-zero consumption (part 2). The dependent variable is log transformed to remove the skewness of the distribution, and the predicted values of log consumption are then retransformed using the smearing estimator.[18] The advantage of using a TPM is that the probability of using health care services and the level of health services consumed for consumers are described by different functions as it is most likely not the same mechanisms that determine the barriers of starting to consume as the amount of health care consumed for people who are already consumers.

---

[50] In the literature the terms 'direct' and 'indirect' standardization are used in different ways. Here the approach from Gravelle is used.

To approximate a linear model, partial effects for each of the variables included in the TPM were estimated using treatment effects. For each of the dummy variables the average partial effects were computed for the respondents who possessed the characteristic.[4,20] For the continuous variables the average effects were computed by approximating the slope by predicting consumption for the observed values with small numbers added and subtracted to these values.[4]

To draw inference on the regression models and the augmented partial concentration indices the non-parametric bootstrap method was used with 1000 replications. The bootstrap method was adapted to reflect the stratified sampling with respect to municipalities. Within each municipality a 1000 resampled data sets were constructed with the sizes of the original municipal sample sizes. Adding the data sets from each of the municipalities together resulted in 1000 stratified resampled data sets. With such a large number of replications a few resampled data sets had "extreme" observations such as categorical variables with empty categories (17 resampled data sets could not be used). The bootstrapping was carried out for a little more than 1000 replications and the first 1000 usable resamples were used. All computations were repeated on each of the resampled data sets and the variability was used to obtain standard errors and confidence limits.

Results

Table 1 shows descriptive statistics and concentration indices and t-statistics for aggregate health care and for each of the health care sectors. Mean aggregate health care is estimated to DKK 18,102 for the two year period. The concentration index for aggregate health care utilization is estimated to -0.136 and is statistical significant indicating that health care is concentrated among the lower income groups. The biggest contributor is hospital visits with 64 percent of aggregate health care, and the concentration index for hospital visits constitute about 90 percent of the index value. The concentration indices for GP services and prescription medicine indicate that GP services and prescription medicine are also distributed unevenly with a concentration among the lower income groups. Dental treatments on the other hand are concentrated among the higher income groups. The concentration indices for physiotherapy and specialist treatment are not statistically significant.

Table 1. Descriptive statistics and concentration indices of aggregate health care and in each of the health care sectors

	Mean(DKK)[a]	Std (DKK)	C	t-value[b]	weight	contrib	contribpct
Hospital	11502	47490	-0.191	-4.33	0.635	-0.121	89.353
GP	1639	1826	-0.105	-8.94	0.091	-0.010	7.012
Physio	395	2243	-0.052	-0.86	0.022	-0.001	0.836
Specialist	578	1732	-0.048	-1.49	0.032	-0.002	1.127
Dentist	1680	1537	0.102	10.61	0.093	0.009	-6.969
Medicine	2307	5399	-0.092	-3.68	0.127	-0.012	8.641
Aggregate	18102	50079	-0.136	-4.60	1.000	-0.136	100.000

Notes: Data weighted by the reciprocals of their selection probabilities.
[a]Health care costs for a two year period, Denmark Kroner.
[b]t-statistics from the regression model (formula 1).

Table 2 shows descriptive statistics, concentration indices and t-statistics for each of the explanatory variables from the regression analysis shown in formula (2). The concentration index applied on income reduces the index to a Gini-coefficient. However, to follow the practice from the literature the natural logarithm has been taken of income to reduce the skewness of the income distribution, and the concentration index then represents the Gini-coefficient of the logarithm of income. Income inequality is one source of income-related inequality in health care utilization. Males and females aged 31-45 and 46-60 are significantly better off than the rest of the age groups with respect to income, while males and females aged 61-70 and 71-80 are significantly worse off than the rest of the age groups indicating that income is highest for the middle aged.

Low education (short or no education) is distributed among the lower income classes whereas medium education (post secondary education but not university degree) is distributed more amongst the higher income classes. With respect to occupational status, the skilled workers, white-collar workers and self-employed are distributed among the higher income classes, whereas the rest of the occupational groups are distributed among the lower income groups.

When it comes to the lifestyle variables the concentration indices for smoking and excessive alcohol consumption are not statistical significant (but present the expected signs, however). Daily consumption of raw vegetables is distributed among the higher income groups, and daily consumption of fruit and a lifestyle without physical exercises are distributed among the lower income classes.

The concentration index for health status (the EQ score) is positive and significant indicating that good health is concentrated among the higher income classes.

Table 2. Descriptive statistics and concentration indices for each of the 36 explanatory variables

	Mean[a]	std	C	t-value[b]
ln(income)	11.986	0.770	0.034	135.35
Male (31-45)	0.147	0.354	0.462	19.03
Male (46-60)	0.149	0.356	0.436	17.96
Male (61-70)	0.057	0.231	-0.088	-2.03
Male (71-80)	0.032	0.176	-0.286	-4.87
Female (16-30)	0.110	0.313	-0.481	-16.52
Female (31-45)	0.157	0.364	0.089	3.61
Female (46-60)	0.124	0.329	0.014	0.50
Female (61-70)	0.062	0.240	-0.426	-10.37
Female (71-80)	0.036	0.187	-0.508	-9.35
Low education	0.650	0.477	-0.008	-1.06
Medium education	0.148	0.355	0.327	13.13
Other education	0.138	0.345	-0.576	-23.51
Skilledworker	0.145	0.353	0.237	9.29
White-collarworker	0.307	0.461	0.347	23.61
Selfemployed	0.043	0.203	0.555	11.25
Assisting spouse	0.005	0.069	-0.192	-1.24
Housewife	0.014	0.118	-0.607	-6.86
Apprentice	0.015	0.122	-0.551	-6.41
Student	0.103	0.305	-0.708	-24.72
Retired	0.188	0.391	-0.371	-17.54
Unemployed	0.021	0.144	-0.338	-4.67
Other job	0.061	0.240	0.119	2.84
Cohabitant	0.146	0.354	0.063	2.43
Separated	0.007	0.085	0.129	1.03
Divorced	0.053	0.224	0.079	1.74
Widowed	0.047	0.212	-0.321	-6.72
Alone	0.192	0.394	-0.374	-17.99
Other	0.002	0.042	0.138	0.54
Daily smoker	0.357	0.479	-0.022	-1.54
High alcohol	0.103	0.304	0.023	0.72
Vegetables, cooked	0.294	0.456	0.022	1.34
Vegetables, raw	0.286	0.452	0.048	2.83
Fruit	0.595	0.491	-0.011	-1.21
No exercises	0.103	0.305	-0.069	-2.18
EQ score	0.896	0.155	0.013	7.35

Notes: Weighted by the reciprocals of their selection probabilities
[a]Max,min for ln(income): (10.127,13.561) for EQ score: (-0.266,1) for all other variables: (0,1)
[b]t-statistics from the regression model (formula 1)

In Table 3 the average partial effects are shown for all the explanatory variables for each of the seven TPMs. The TPMs can be interpreted as reduced form demand functions for health care. For (log of) income the partial effects are positive and significant only for dental services and aggregate health care. For the rest of the sectors the partial effects are statistically insignificant at a 5 percent level of significance.

Table 3. Partial effects of the two-part-models for health care consumption

	Hospital	GP	Physiotherapy	Specialist	Dentist	Medicine	Aggregate
ln(income)	859.8	-10.3	136.6*	89.3*	342.4***	55.1	1908.5**
Male (31-45)	-2284.4	17.6	-13.2	1.3	200.7	236.5**	-638.8
Male (46-60)	-497.8	-32.2	-180.6	67.5	709.2***	1610.5***	3147.7*
Male (61-70)	4655.0	341.7	66.7	190.6	453.6**	3794.6***	6160.3
Male (71-80)	18610.6*	1371.0***	-88.8	251.9	-11.2	7382.6***	21893.3***
Female (16-30)	3552.7*	1401.5***	28.2	181.7***	52.3	336.4***	5798.8***
Female (31-45)	-977.0	738.0***	-11.2	140.2	422.8***	745.2***	4283.3***
Female (46-60)	-2386.8	743.8***	177.9	246.2**	873.7***	3262.8***	8750.3***
Female (61-70)	-10767.1	791.5***	237.7	260.1*	459.1***	6789.1***	9051.8**
Female (71-80)	-989.7	1949.8***	769.2	958.1***	121.9	10922.1***	30712.8***
Low education	-1819.0	50.0	-81.7	-115.7	193.4	-1018.3	-335.4
Medium education	-2856.7	-131.3	100.8	-165.6	317.0*	-981.1*	-816.5
Other education	-4189.5	75.4	-298.9	-157.0	171.1	-637.3	-1377.3
Skilled worker	-98.4	-17.1	73.7	-216.4***	-58.3	-86.4	149.7
White-collar worker	639.3	-87.6	105.8	-108.6	-20.6	35.2	484.7
Selfemployed	4306.6	-78.9	216.4	-58.4	183.0	-112.1	3052.9
Assisting spouse	-2011.0	-877.1	700.5	-396.1	-74.6	-1705.6*	-5291.6
Housewife	6336.3	439.2	319.5	233.0	647.0*	2282.6	9385.6*
Apprentice	3284.9	160.1	404.6	210.7	-25.2	298.3	3428.3
Student	682.8	-188.4	82.4	0.5	-59.4	164.8	-5.1
Retired	19912.9***	250.4	518.5***	36.5	-3.0	3025.7***	14442.8***
Unemployed	11685.9	520.8	435.9	-27.9	309.5	1908.1*	14459.9**
Other job	5219.4*	-159.0	116.6	13.3	-4.6	-249.4	3343.0
Cohabitant	-1959.3	-38.5	-37.0	-114.5	-105.7	-313.0***	-2226.2**
Separated	-7035.8	1022.8*	250.8	-61.5	-593.5*	-1349.1	-5131.9
Divorced	5716.0	332.9	-458.0*	-101.8	-43.9	541.6	4156.6
Widowed	-7440.7	237.9	-676.2**	-387.1**	26.7	114.4	-5920.6
Alone	-2310.7	-122.1	48.8	-85.2	-247.0***	-75.2	-2941.2***
Other	-10074.8**	618.8	-530.1***	-553.7***	-609.1	-110.9	-5797.5
Daily smoker	1203.8	5.0	-86.6	-91.2	-70.6	-547.5**	-725.3
High alcohol	-821.8	-233.8**	-76.5	-49.4	-1.5	310.6	724.0
Vegetables, cooked	1322.9	160.4*	-88.4	-1.9	-11.2	472.3	1709.1
Vegetables, raw	1866.5	70.6	23.2	87.6	64.4	24.6	1811.6*
Fruit	4761.8***	225.8***	-34.0	58.2	109.8	451.8*	4682.8***
No exercises	1884.1	89.3	153.4	-21.1	-211.9*	727.3	1771.5
EQ score	-33593.7***	-3290.0***	-1529.8***	-912.0***	-584.5***	-7067.7***	-47976.1***

Notes: Bootstrapped SE to indicate significance.
***Indicates coefficient estimates significantly different from zero at the 1 percent level.
**Indicates coefficient estimates significantly different from zero at the 5 percent level.
*Indicates coefficient estimates significantly different from zero at the 10 percent level.

Age and gender are important in some of the sectors. For aggregate health care women consume statistically more than the reference group of male 16-30. This effect is increased for the higher age groups. The pattern is similar for prescription medicine and GP visits. For hospital contacts, however, age and gender do not seem to matter in a model when health status is controlled for.

Education, marital status and occupational status are of little importance with the exception of being retired, which does have a positive influence on health care utilization in some of the sectors.

The life style variables like smoking and alcohol consumption do not seem to have an influence on health care consumption as could have been expected. However, their influence probably works through a lower health status, which is controlled for by the EQ-5D score. The partial effect of the EQ-5D score is negative and significant for aggregate health and for all the health care sectors at a 1 percent level of significance.

Tabel 4. Decomposition of C: Contribution from each health care sector and explanatory variable in percent of predicted concentration index[a]

	Hospital	GP	Physiotherapy	Specialist	Dentist	Medicine	Aggregate
ln(income)	18.14	-0.22	2.88*	1.88*	7.23***	1.16	31.08
Male (31-45)	-7.95	0.06	-0.05	0.00	0.70	0.82**	-6.41
Male (46-60)	-1.65	-0.11	-0.60	0.22	2.35***	5.34***	5.56
Male (61-70)	-1.19	-0.09	-0.02	-0.05	-0.12	-0.97*	-2.44
Male (71-80)	-8.68	-0.64***	0.04	-0.12	0.01	-3.44***	-12.84**
Female (16-30)	-9.60*	-3.79***	-0.08	-0.49**	-0.14	-0.91***	-15.01***
Female (31-45)	-0.70	0.53***	-0.01	0.10	0.30***	0.53***	0.76
Female (46-60)	-0.22	0.07	0.02	0.02	0.08	0.29	0.26
Female (61-70)	14.41	-1.06***	-0.32	-0.35*	-0.61***	-9.08***	2.98
Female (71-80)	0.93	-1.84***	-0.73	-0.90**	-0.11	-10.30***	-12.95
Low education	0.50	-0.01	0.02	0.03	-0.05	0.28	0.77
Medium education	-7.09	-0.33	0.25	-0.41	0.79*	-2.43*	-9.22
Other education	17.05	-0.31	1.22	0.64	-0.70	2.59	20.49
Skilled worker	-0.17	-0.03	0.13	-0.38***	-0.10	-0.15	-0.71
White-collar worker	3.49	-0.48	0.58	-0.59	-0.11	0.19	3.08
Selfemployed	5.27	-0.10	0.26	-0.07	0.22	-0.14	5.45
Assisting spouse	0.09	0.04	-0.03	0.02	0.00	0.08	0.20
Housewife	-2.79	-0.19	-0.14	-0.10	-0.28*	-1.00	-4.51
Apprentice	-1.39	-0.07	-0.17	-0.09	0.01	-0.13	-1.84
Student	-2.56	0.71	-0.31	0.00	0.22	-0.62	-2.56
Retired	-71.06***	-0.89	-1.85***	-0.13	0.01	-10.8***	-84.72***
Unemployed	-4.29	-0.19	-0.16	0.01	-0.11	-0.70*	-5.44
Other job	1.95	-0.06	0.04	0.00	0.00	-0.09	1.84
Cohabitant	-0.92	-0.02	-0.02	-0.05	-0.05	-0.15*	-1.20
Separated	-0.33	0.05	0.01	0.00	-0.03	-0.06	-0.37
Divorced	1.21	0.07	-0.10	-0.02	-0.01	0.12	1.27
Widowed	5.76	-0.18	0.52**	0.30**	-0.02	-0.09	6.29
Alone	8.50	0.45	-0.18	0.31	0.91***	0.28	10.27
Other	-0.13	0.01	-0.01	-0.01	-0.01	0.00	-0.14
Daily smoker	-0.49	0.00	0.03	0.04	0.03	0.22	-0.17
High alcohol	-0.10	-0.03	-0.01	-0.01	0.00	0.04	-0.10
Vegetables, cooked	0.44	0.05	-0.03	0.00	0.00	0.16	0.62
Vegetables, raw	1.30	0.05	0.02	0.06	0.04	0.02	1.49
Fruit	-1.55	-0.07	0.01	-0.02	-0.04	-0.15	-1.81
No exercises	-0.68	-0.03	-0.06	0.01	0.08	-0.26	-0.95
EQ score	-20.76***	-2.03***	-0.95***	-0.56***	-0.36***	-4.37***	-29.04***
Pred.CI	-65.25***	-10.68***	0.25	-0.71	10.11***	-33.72***	-100.00***

Notes: Bootstrapped SE to indicate significance.
[a]The contributions have been multiplied by -1 to maintain the original signs of the contributions.
***Indicates coefficient estimates significantly different from zero at the 1 percent level.
**Indicates coefficient estimates significantly different from zero at the 5 percent level.
*Indicates coefficient estimates significantly different from zero at the 10 percent level.

The overall decomposition of the concentration index is presented in Table 4. Summing all the contributions from different sectors and various explanatory variables result in the predicted concentration index. This is equivalent to the first four terms on the right hand side of formula 5. The generalized concentration index is estimated as the residual term (the difference between the observed and predicted concentration index). The generalized concentration index is relatively small as most of the inequality is explained by the explanatory variables. However, for some of the health care sectors the generalized concentration is rather big. One reason for this is that the generalized concentration index consists of unexplained variation as well as the approximation error from the linear approximation. Positive contributions increase the size of the inequality and negative contributions decrease the size of inequality (or increase inequality in favor of the lower income groups). The biggest contributors to the concentration index come from (log of) income, health status and being retired.

Tabel 5. Decomposition of C: Contribution from each health care sector and explanatory variable

	Hospital	GP	Physiotherapy	Specialist	Dentist	Medicine	Aggregate
Decompositions in each sector separately							
Income	0.031	-0.003	0.143*	0.064*	0.084***	0.010	0.034
Need	-0.060*	-0.106***	-0.132***	-0.072***	0.024***	-0.187***	-0.075***
Socio-econ	-0.080***	-0.018	0.003	-0.018	0.008	-0.109***	-0.066***
Lifestyle	-0.002	0.000	-0.001	0.003	0.001	0.000	-0.001
Error	-0.080*	0.022*	-0.064	-0.024	-0.016*	0.194***	-0.028
Obs. C	-0.191***	-0.105***	-0.052	-0.048	0.102***	-0.092***	-0.136***
HI	-0.131***	0.001	0.080	0.024	0.078***	0.095***	-0.061*
Weighted by contribution							
Income	0.020	0.000	0.003*	0.002*	0.008***	0.001	0.034
Need	-0.038*	-0.01***	-0.003***	-0.002***	0.002***	-0.024***	-0.075***
Socio-econ	-0.051***	-0.002	0.000	-0.001	0.001	-0.014***	-0.066***
Lifestyle	-0.001	0.000	0.000	0.000	0.000	0.000	-0.001
Error	-0.051*	0.002*	-0.001	-0.001	-0.001*	0.025***	-0.028
Obs. C	-0.121***	-0.010***	-0.001	-0.002	0.009***	-0.012***	-0.136***
HI	-0.083***	0.000	0.002	0.001	0.007***	0.012***	-0.061*

Notes: Bootstrapped SE to indicate significance.
***Indicates coefficient estimates significantly different from zero at the 1 percent level.
**Indicates coefficient estimates significantly different from zero at the 5 percent level.
*Indicates coefficient estimates significantly different from zero at the 10 percent level.

In Table 5 the contributions are categorized into types of variables according to formula 2. The need based variables consist of the age and gender dummies and the EQ-5D health status variable. The HI index is estimated as all the categories added together excluding the need variables, but including the error term (the generalized concentration index). Bootstrapping standard errors have been computed to indicate statistical signifance. When standardizing for need, the income-related inequality for aggregate health care is no longer statistically significant. However, for prescription medicine and dentistry significant inequality in favor of the higher income groups emerges, and in the hospital sector we see that the inequality in favor of the lower income groups is still significant. As could be expected (log of) income contributes positively to income-related inequality. However, this is not the case for GP services where income contributes negatively. Except for dental treatments the need based variables exhibit a negative contribution to inequality in all health sectors. That is, controlling for need the size of the inequality diminishes. The socio-economic variables and life style variables contribute positively in some sectors and negatively in others, and there is no clear pattern.

Discussion

For this study a health survey was merged with various individual level computerized registers to give a more precise measure of health care consumption than the self-reported number of visits you often find in health surveys. The analysis showed that the income groups consume a bigger share the health care services than the higher income groups. After standardization for age, gender and health status there is no significant horizontal inequity for aggregate health care use at a 5 percent level of significance. This suggests that the Danish health care system is not in general inequitable in terms of horizontal inequity. In two sectors, however, a different picture emerges. For specific types of care the least advantaged have a lower share of the prescription medicine and dental treatments than expected. In the hospital sector, on the other hand, the need based variables cannot explain the high concentration of hospital treatment among the lower income groups.

The decomposition analysis showed that health care inequality is a diversified matter, and an overall measure of income-related inequality may be too crude to measure health care inequality for specific purposes. Policies combating inequalities in health care might not show any changes in the overall index if decreases in inequality in one type of health care are offset by increases in another. Therefore, it is relevant to know the sources of health care inequality.

Lifestyle variables were included as explanatory variables in this study as it is well documented that smoking, alcohol habits, and diet and activity patterns have a big influence on health.[21-24] The life style variables, however, did not seem to contribute significantly to inequality, at least not directly. Although lifestyle behavior is sometimes rooted in firmly cemented cultural habits, the possibilities of health policy initiatives might still have better chances of altering lifestyles than socio-economic and socio-demographic conditions.

In van Doorslaer et al. health care services are measured by the number of visits extracted from household surveys in 21 OECD countries.[3] They found significant pro-poor income-related inequality in inpatient hospital care and GP visits in Denmark. When standardizing for need the inequality vanished for hospital care, but not for GP visits, whereas in the present study the inequality vanished for GP visits but not for hospital care. For dental visits there is agreement between the two studies. Both found income-related inequality in dental care in favor of the higher income groups, with or without standardization. For specialist treatment there is a serious deviation between this study and other studies. The present study found no significant inequality in specialist care. When standardizing for need significant inequality for specialist treatment is found in most countries, including Denmark.

The survey data made it possible to gather information on variables, like self-perceived health status that can normally not be found in registers. The use of survey data, however, limited the size of the population, which could have been considerably bigger, had the data only consisted of registers. The use of survey data also caused non-response. The non-response analysis suggested that the non-respondents had a higher level of health care consumption than respondents. The survey data were gathered through telephone interviews. This means that people too weak to have a telephone conversation obviously are not included in the study. This could be one explanation for the higher level of health care consumption among the non-respondents for most types of health care. The income variable was taken from the health survey. Income is a sensitive question and a large fraction of the respondents were reluctant to answer that question. 485 respondents were left out of the analysis due to missing observations with respect to income[51].

The study covers only somatic hospital treatment and services that are subject to partial or complete reimbursement by the Public Health Insurance. For most types of health care there is no co-payment (although private for-profit supply of some health care services does exist). For dentistry, however, a considerable share of the services is not reimbursed at all, and these services are not included in the database. If income-related inequalities exist they are most likely bigger for the kind of services the patients have to pay for. Therefore, the concentration index for dentistry is certainly a conservative estimate.

For medicine only prescription medicine in the primary health care sector entitled to reimbursement is in the database. In addition, prescription medicine bought from pharmacies outside Funen County, medicine used in hospitals, and illegal purchases of medicine over the internet are not covered by the database either (medicine used in hospitals is included in hospital charges).

The health care data were limited to two years (2000 and 2001). The longer the period is, the smaller is the problem of zero consumption data and random fluctuations. However, the health status indicators are point estimates, and will be less valid as standardization variables for health care consumption taken place too long before or after the time of the interview.

As a proxy for need for health care EQ-5D values were used. Health status as a proxy for need for health care services is common in the literature.[2,3,25,26] Health status is not always a good proxy for need for health care. Some products are taken for the preventive effect. Furthermore, when treatment cures the illnesses the need for health care is not accounted for by the health status indicators, which might show good or perfect health as a result of the treatment. For dental care the health status variables seem to be particular inappropriate as general health status cannot be expected a good proxy for dental health status. If preferable the EQ score could be excluded from the need component in formula 6.

---

[51] The income variable from the health survey has been validated against income from national registers and there are no signs of important differences between the observed income and the income from registers.

Conclusion

The decomposition approach suggests that health care is in general equally distributed in Denmark when need based variables are controlled for. The overall result is a consequence of a number of off-setting effects from different types of health care and a complicated pattern of various explanatory variables. The analyses show that decompositions can be useful when using concentration indices to estimate income-related inequality in health care. Different health care sectors contribute to inequality in aggregate health care to a varying degree. Therefore, decompositions contribute with information about the importance of the different health care sectors and off-setting effects, that would otherwise have been missed in the aggregate data.

Acknowledgments

The authors would like to thank Funen County for delivery of hospital data and OPED for delivery of prescription records. The study was carried out thanks to a research grant from The Health Insurance Foundation, Denmark (Sygekassernes Helsefond). The authors alone are responsible for the contents of the article.

References

1. van Doorslaer E, Wagstaff A, Calonge S, Christiansen T, Gerfin M, Gottschalk P, Janssen R, Lachaud C, Leu RE, Nolan B, O'donnell O, Paci P, Pereira j, Pinto CG, Propper C, Reñé J, Rochaix L, Rodríguez M, Rutten F, Upward R, Wolfe B. Equity in the delivery of health care: some international comparisons. *J Health Econ* 1992;**11**:389-411.

2. van Doorslaer E, Wagstaff A, van der Burg H, Christiansen T, De Graeve D, Duchesne I, Gerdtham UG, Gerfin M, Geurts J, Gross L, Häkkinen U, John J, Klavus J, Leu RE, Nolan B, O'Donnell O, Propper C, Puffer F, Schellhorn M, Sundberg G, Winkelhake O. Equity in the delivery of health care in Europe and the US. *J Health Econ* 2000;**19**:553-83.

3. van Doorslaer E, Masseria, C, the OECD Health Equity Research Group Members. Income-Related Inequality in the Use of Medical Care in 21 OECD Countries. 14. 2004. Paris, OECD. OECD Health working papers.

4. van Doorslaer E, Koolman X, Jones AM. Explaining income-related inequalities in doctor utilisation in Europe. *Health Econ* 2004;**13**:629-47.

5. van Doorslaer E, Koolman X. Explaining the differences in income-related health inequalities across European countries. *Health Econ* 2004;**13**:609-28.

6. Wagstaff A, van Doorslaer E, Watanabe N. On Decomposing the Causes of Health Sector Inequalities with an Application to Malnutrition Inequalities in Vietnam. *J Econometrics* 2003;**112**:207-23.

7. Clarke PM, Gerdtham UG, Connelly LB. A note on the decomposition of the health concentration index. *Health Econ* 2003;**12**:511-16.

8. Gravelle H. Measuring income related inequality in health: standardisation and the partial concentration index. *Health Econ* 2003;**12**:803-19.

9. Culyer AJ. Health, Health Expenditures and Equity. In: van Doorslaer E, Wagstaff A, Rutten F, editors. Equity in the Finance and Delivery of Health Care: An International Perspective. Oxford University Press, 1993.

10. Lauridsen J, Christiansen T, Gundgaard J, Häkkinen U, Sintonen H. Decomposition of socio-economic determination of income-related health inequality by health domains. Forthcoming 2005.

11. Gundgaard J, Sørensen J. . Evaluering af Fyns Amts Forebyggelsesstrategi: Baseline survey om sundhedstilstand og adfærd omkring tobak, alcohol, kost og motion [Evaluation of the Prevention Strategy in Funen County: Baseline Survey on Behaviour with respct to Tobacco, Alcohol, Diet and Exercise]. 2002. Funen County.

12. Hallas J. Conducting pharmacoepidemiologic research in Denmark. *Pharmacoepidemiol Drug Safe* 2001;**10**:619-23.

13. Brooks R. Quality of life measures. *Crit Care Med* 1996;**24**:1769.

14. Brooks R. EuroQol: the current state of play. *Health Policy* 1996;**37**:53-72.

15. Dolan P. Modeling valuations for EuroQol health states. *Med Care* 1997;**35**:1095-108.

16. Wittrup-Jensen KU, Lauridsen JT, Gudex C, Brooks R, and Pedersen KM. Estimating Danish EQ-5D tariffs using the time trade-off (TTO) and visual analogue scale (VAS) methods. In Norinder AL, Pedersen KM, Roos P (eds) Proceedings of the 18th Plenary Meeting of the EuroQol Group, 6th - 7th September, 2001, Copenhagen, Denmark, IHE- The Swedish Institute for Health Economics, Lund. 2001.

17. Kakwani N, Wagstaff A, van Doorslaer E. Socioeconomic Inequalities in Health: Measurement, Computation, and Statistical Inference. *J Econometrics* 1997;**77**:87-103.

18. Manning WG. The logged dependent variable, heteroscedasticity, and the retransformation problem. *J Health Econ* 1998;**17**:283-95.

19. Lipscomb J, Ancukiewicz M, Parmigiani G, Hasselblad V, Samsa G, Matchar DB. Predicting the cost of illness: a comparison of alternative models applied to stroke. *Med Decis Making* 1998;**18**:S39-S56.

20. Wooldridge JM. Econometric Analysis of Cross Section and Panel Data. The MIT Press, 2002.

21. Ferrucci L, Izmirlian G, Leveille S et al. Smoking, physical activity, and active life expectancy. *Am J Epidemiol* 1999;**149**:645-53.

22. McGinnis JM, Foege WH. Actual causes of death in the United States. *JAMA* 1993;**270**:2207-12.

23. Oguma Y, Sesso HD, Paffenbarger RS, Jr., Lee IM. Physical activity and all cause mortality in women: a review of the evidence. *Br J Sports Med* 2002;**36**:162-72.

24. Paffenbarger RS Jr, Hyde RT, Wing AL, Lee IM, Jung DL, Kampert JB. The association of changes in physical-activity level

and other lifestyle characteristics with mortality among men. *N Engl J Med* 1993;**328**:538-45.

25. van der Meer JB, van den Bos J, Mackenbach JP. Socioeconomic differences in the utilization of health services in a Dutch population: the contribution of health status. *Health Policy* 1996;**37**:1-18.

26. Van der Heyden JH, Demarest S, Tafforeau J, Van Oyen H. Socio-economic differences in the utilisation of health services in Belgium. *Health Policy* 2003;**65**:153-65.

Chapter 5

A decomposition of income-related health inequality applied to EQ-5D

Jens Gundgaard, Jørgen Lauridsen

European Journal of Health Economics 2006; 7: 231-237

Abstract

Income-related inequality in health and its relationship to socio-demographic characteristics have received considerable attention in the health economic literature. Recently, a method was suggested for decomposing income-related health inequality to contributions from individual characteristics via additive dimensions, and this was applied to a Finnish case based on 15D health scores, where health is considered to be a sum of 15 individual health dimensions. The present study adds to this literature in several ways. First, we apply the decomposition approach to a Danish case which can be benchmarked to the Finnish. Second, we show how to apply the methodology to EQ-5D scores, which deviate from 15D scores by expressing health as individual depreciations of an equal endowment of perfect health. Third, we add life style factors to the determinants of income-related health inequality. The empirical part of the study reveals discrepancies which can be attributed to differences between Finland and Denmark and to differences between the construction of 15D and EQ-5D scores. Finally, evidence of impact of life style factors on income-related health inequality is found.

Keywords: EQ-5D, Health status index, Concentration index, Inequality, Decomposition

Introduction

Health-related quality-of-life (HRQL) measures are frequently used in health policy decision making to allocate health care resources efficiently. However, policy-makers are not only concerned about efficiency. The distribution of health in the population is also of concern. Equality in health is among the main objectives of health policy in many countries.[1-3] This implies that HRQL measures are also applied in studies of equality in health. Income-related inequality in health is measured by the concentration index, which has become a standard method for measuring health inequalities.[4-8] The concentration index summarizes income-related inequality as a single measure. However, as the HRQL instrument consists of various dimensions of health, it can be useful to decompose the concentration index into different components in order to understand the sources that contribute to inequality in health.[9] Furthermore, if health is related to determinants such as socioeconomic and sociodemographic characteristics and life style factors, the concentration index can also be decomposed into contributions from background characteristics.[10] For policy purposes it is relevant to be informed about relationships between characteristics and health inequality to be able to target policies optimally.

The present study considers the EQ-5D instrument which is frequently used in cost-effectiveness analyses or in health surveys to assess HRQL. The EQ-5D questionnaire is a standardized generic health instrument consisting of five dimensions of health: mobility, self-care, usual activities, pain/discomfort, and anxiety/depression. Each dimension is divided into three levels of health: no problems, some or moderate problems, or extreme problems.[11-14] The Danish EQ-5D, established by Wittrup-Jensen et al. [15], implicitly added a sixth dimension consisting of an indicator for being dysfunctional (i.e. having moderate or severe problems in any of the five dimensions). The six dimensions are summarized into a single HRQL index by weighting the levels of the dimensions by a standard set of general population preference time trade-off (TTO) weights.[16-18]

The analyses of the study follow the lines of earlier studies [9,10,19]. Clark et al. [9] decomposed a concentration index by dimension and subgroup separately and Wagstaff et al. [10] used a multivariate regression approach. The regression approach assisted a decomposition of the single characteristic's impact on inequality in a health component into (a) its regressive impact on the variation in the health component and (b) the impact due to income-related inequality in the characteristic itself.[10] Lauridsen et al. [19] merged the decomposition by dimension from Clark et al. [9] with the regression approach from Wagstaff et al.[10] This was applied on a concentration index with health status measured by the generic health instrument 15D.[20] The concentration index was decomposed into the different dimensions of health summing up to the index and the effect on health from different socioeconomic characteristics. Lauridsen et al. [19] applied the decomposition on data from a Finnish survey. The analysis showed that the different components of health contributed to health and inequality in health to varying degree, and that relationships to socioeconomic and sociodemographic characteristics varied considerably.

Method

Health status was measured using Danish EQ-5D TTO values.[15] In addition to coefficients for the five dimensions of the EQ-5D instrument, the Danish TTO model includes an indicator for any dysfunctional state (i.e. having moderate or severe problems in any of the five dimensions). This indicator was treated as a sixth dimension.[15] As with most generic HRQL measures [21], the EQ-5D comprises dimensions that represent different aspects of health. For several indices the final health status measure is calculated as a sum of scores for each dimension, i.e. as:

$$Y = \sum_{j=1}^{J} Y_j, \qquad (1)$$

where Y_j is the contribution to overall health from dimension j. The EQ-5D fits into this frame, as it can be written as:

$$Y = 1 + \sum_{j=1}^{J} Y_j = \sum_{j=0}^{J} Y_j, \qquad (2)$$

with $Y_0 = 1$ denoting an endowment of perfect health, and $Y_1, .., Y_6$ measuring depreciations of this endowment (rather than contributions to health) caused by moderate or severe health problems. The concentration index for Y can be decomposed as a weighted average:

$$C = \sum_{j=0}^{J} w_j C_j = \sum_{j=1}^{J} w_j C_j, \qquad (3)$$

where C is the concentration index for Y, C_j the concentration index for Y_j, and w_j a weight attached to the j'th dimension, estimated as $w_j = \frac{\mu_j}{\mu}$, with μ and μ_j being the means of Y and Y_j, respectively. The first equality of Eq. 3 is due to Clark et al. [9], the second follows as C_0 is equal to zero. The concentration index of Y_j with respect to income can be calculated conveniently by applying the regression [10]:

$$2\sigma_j^2 \left(\frac{Y_j}{\mu} \right) = \alpha_j + \beta_j R + \varepsilon_j, \qquad (4)$$

where σ_j^2 is the variance of R and

$$R = \frac{r - 0.5}{n} \qquad (5)$$

is the fractional income rank of the n individuals, with r being the unconditional income rank. The estimate of C_j is then equal to the OLS coefficient of the relative rank, $\hat{\beta}_j$, and approximate standard errors and t values are easily obtained from standard statistical packages.

For the purpose of decomposing C by socioeconomic and life style determinants it is assumed that each health component Y_j ($j = 1, ..., J$) is linked to K regressors through a linear regression:

$$Y_j = \tau_j + \sum_{k=1}^{K} \delta_{jk} x_k + \varepsilon_j. \qquad (6)$$

Following the approach of Wagstaff et al. [10] and given the relationship between health and the determinants the concentration index can be decomposed into contributions from the regressors as

$$C_j = \sum_{k=1}^{K} \frac{\delta_{jk} \mu_k}{\mu_j} C_k + \frac{2}{\mu_j n} \sum_{i=1}^{n} \varepsilon_{j(i)} R_{(i)} = \sum_{k=1}^{K} \eta_{jk} C_k + \frac{1}{\mu_j} CG_{\varepsilon_j}. \qquad (7)$$

where μ_k and C_k are the mean and concentration index of the k'th regressor. Applying (3), the decomposition of C follows as in Lauridsen et al.[19]

$$C = \sum_{j=1}^{6} w_j C_j = \sum_{j=1}^{J} w_j [\sum_{k=1}^{K} \frac{\delta_{jk}\mu_k}{\mu_j} C_k + \frac{1}{\mu_j} CG_{\varepsilon_j}]$$

$$= \sum_{j=1}^{J} \sum_{k=1}^{K} \frac{\delta_{jk}\mu_k}{\mu} C_k + \sum_{j=1}^{J} \frac{1}{\mu} CG_{\varepsilon_j} \qquad (8)$$

$$= C^{PRED} + CG^{RESID}$$

As demonstrated by Lauridsen et al. [19], the contribution from the k'th regressor to C^{PRED} is then obtained as

$$\sum_{j=1}^{J} \frac{\delta_{jk}\mu_k}{\mu} C_k, \qquad (9)$$

while the contribution from the j'th dimension is obtained as

$$\sum_{k=1}^{K} \frac{\delta_{jk}\mu_k}{\mu} C_k. \qquad (10)$$

Data

5,000 persons living in the county of Funen, Denmark, aged 16-80 years were drawn from The Centralised Civil Register to participate in a health survey on health status, health behavior and socioeconomic background.[22] The sample was stratified with respect to municipalities, such that small and large municipalities would be represented. Within municipalities the respondents were drawn randomly.[22] The county of Funen is situated right in the middle of Denmark, makes up a little less than 10% of the national population, and is considered representative of the Danes.[23] The data were gathered through telephone interviews that took place in the period from October 2000 through April 2001. An external response rate of 68% was obtained.[22] A number of the respondents did not answer all questions relevant for the present study and had to be excluded, leaving a final working sample of 2,915, or 58%.

Descriptive response/nonresponse analysis was carried out by Gundgaard et al. [22] to shed some light on potential differences between the participants and the nonparticipants. It was found that the number of women and men were approximately equal in the working sample. The participants were on average slightly younger than the nonparticipants. Dividing the respondents into age groups showed that the middle-aged are slightly more prone to participate than the younger or older groups.[22] Income was defined as previous year's gross income (gross of tax and deductibles) and measured as a categorical variable with 17 categories. The respondents were ranked according to their income category. Within the categories the respondents were ranked randomly. Descriptive statistics (means and standard deviations) of the data applied are provided as part of Tables 1 and 2.

Results

Table 1 shows concentration indices and their t statistics for each of the six dimensions of EQ-5D and the overall EQ-5D scores according to Eq. 4. The average overall EQ-5D score is 0.898, and the corresponding concentration index for the EQ-5D score is estimated to 0.013 indicating that health is concentrated among the higher income groups. The scores for the six dimensions express reductions in health rather than contributions to health. The dimensions with the highest mean reductions in health are Pain/discomfort and Dysfunctional with mean scores of -0.0284 and -0.0455, respectively. All the partial EQ-5D indices are negative and statistically significant indicating that ill-health is concentrated among the lower income groups. The weight of each component and the contribution from each component's inequality to the inequality of the overall EQ-5D score is reported according to the decomposition in Eq. 3. Inequality in favor of the higher income groups is most pronounced for Pain/discomfort and Dysfunctional, and these dimensions are also the most contributing factors to overall inequality.

Further, Table 2 shows concentration indices and t statistics for each of the regressors. Both men and women aged 31-45 and 46-60 years are significantly better off than the rest of the age groups with respect to income. Men and women aged 61-70 and 71-80 years are significantly worse off than the rest of the age groups, indicating that income is highest for the middle aged. Low education is distributed among the lower income groups whereas medium education is distributed among the higher income groups. With respect to occupational status, the skilled workers, white-collar workers, and self-employed are distributed among the higher income groups, whereas the rest of the occupational groups are distributed among the lower income groups.

Table 1. Descriptive statistics and concentration indices of EQ-5D and each of its dimensions ($n = 2915$)

	Mean	Std	Min	Max	C_i	T	Std C_i	Weight	Contrib.	Contrib. percent
Mobility	-0.0063	0.0234	-0.411	0	-0.1782	-4.5246	0.0394	-0.0071	0.0013	9.6679
Self-care	-0.0022	0.0171	-0.192	0	-0.1920	-2.2660	0.0847	-0.0024	0.0005	3.5476
Usual activity	-0.0078	0.0223	-0.144	0	-0.1847	-6.0407	0.0306	-0.0086	0.0016	12.2566
Pain/discomfort	-0.0284	0.0653	-0.396	0	-0.1241	-5.0629	0.0245	-0.0316	0.0039	30.1516
Anxiety/depression	-0.0119	0.0415	-0.367	0	-0.1471	-3.9543	0.0372	-0.0133	0.0019	14.9847
Dysfunctional	-0.0455	0.0558	-0.114	0	-0.0755	-5.7823	0.0131	-0.0507	0.0038	29.3916
EQ-5D score	0.8980	0.1543	-0.266	1	0.0130	7.1413	0.0018	1.0000	0.0130	100.0000

Table 2. Descriptive statistics and concentration indices of the regressor variables ($n = 2915$)

	Mean	Std	C_i	t-value	Std C_i
ln(income)[a]	11.9890	0.7579	0.0339	133.9107	0.0003
Male (31-45)	0.1479	0.3550	0.4644	19.1842	0.0242
Male (46-60)	0.1479	0.3550	0.4169	17.0172	0.0245
Male (61-70)	0.0587	0.2350	-0.0918	-2.1422	0.0428
Male (71-80)	0.0346	0.1829	-0.3224	-5.7404	0.0562
Female (16-30)	0.1087	0.3114	-0.4816	-16.4338	0.0293
Female (31-45)	0.1585	0.3653	0.0751	3.0523	0.0246
Female (46-60)	0.1286	0.3349	0.0185	0.6630	0.0278
Female (61-70)	0.0631	0.2432	-0.4319	-10.6806	0.0404
Female (71-80)	0.0360	0.1864	-0.5304	-9.7361	0.0545
Low Education	0.6724	0.4694	-0.0134	-1.7962	0.0075
Medium Education	0.1451	0.3523	0.3304	13.0917	0.0252
Other Education	0.1273	0.3333	-0.5637	-21.6787	0.0260
Skilled worker	0.1554	0.3624	0.2314	9.4142	0.0246
White-collar worker	0.2878	0.4528	0.3563	23.0143	0.0155
Selfemployed	0.0491	0.2160	0.4900	10.6001	0.0462
Assisting spouse	0.0051	0.0716	-0.2533	-1.7030	0.1487
Housewife	0.0148	0.1206	-0.5683	-6.5455	0.0868
Apprentice	0.0154	0.1233	-0.5397	-6.3588	0.0849
Student	0.0926	0.2900	-0.7138	-23.1957	0.0308
Retired	0.1918	0.3938	-0.3767	-18.0856	0.0208
Unemployed	0.0216	0.1454	-0.3299	-4.5981	0.0717
Other job	0.0597	0.2370	0.0868	2.0453	0.0424
Cohabitant	0.1479	0.3550	0.0687	2.6785	0.0257
Separated	0.0058	0.0762	0.1189	0.8508	0.1397
Divorced	0.0511	0.2203	0.0579	1.2566	0.0461
Widowed	0.0453	0.2080	-0.3324	-6.8194	0.0487
Alone	0.1808	0.3849	-0.3775	-17.4149	0.0217
Other	0.0017	0.0414	-0.0376	-0.1457	0.2582
Daily smoker	0.3660	0.4818	-0.0184	-1.3094	0.0141
High alcohol	0.0991	0.2989	0.0182	0.5650	0.0323
Vegetables, cooked	0.2985	0.4577	0.0183	1.1177	0.0164
Vegetables, raw	0.2820	0.4500	0.0369	2.1649	0.0171
Fruit	0.5983	0.4903	-0.0176	-2.0053	0.0088
No exercises	0.1142	0.3182	-0.0728	-2.4466	0.0298
Smoker and alcohol	0.0480	0.2139	-0.0284	-0.5954	0.0476
smoke,alco,no exer	0.0099	0.0993	-0.2064	-1.9343	0.1067

[a] Ln(income) ranged from a minimum of 10.1266 to a maximum of 13.5606

Regarding life-style variables the concentration indices for smoking and excessive alcohol consumption are not statistically significant (but present the expected signs, however). Daily consumption of raw vegetables is distributed among the higher income groups, and daily consumption of fruit and a life style without physical exercises are distributed among the lower income groups. As it is obvious that different life style factors may interact with each other, two interaction variables have been constructed: one with smoking and excessive alcohol, and one with smoking, excessive alcohol and no exercises. The concentration indices for these variables are negative indicating that interactions of unhealthy life-style are distributed among the lower income groups. However, the coefficients are not statistically significant.

Table 3 shows coefficients from the regression analyses according to Eq. 6. Income is positively related to the overall EQ-5D score and to the other dimensions and significantly so for the overall EQ-5D score and Dysfunctional ($p<0.05$). For the overall EQ-5D score men aged 31-45 and 46-60 years and women aged 30 or under, 31-45, and 46-60 years are worse off than the reference group of men aged 30 or under. The older age groups do not differ significantly from the reference group. This may indicate that persons learn to cope with their disabilities at old age. Educational level and occupational status do not seem to affect health status. Only the retired and the unemployed seem to have a significantly lower health status than the reference group of unskilled workers. It appears that being active in the labor market is of greater importance than the actual job type. Regarding life-style, daily smoking affects the overall EQ-5D score and the Pain/discomfort and Anxiety/depression dimensions negatively. Another important life-style variable is no exercises, which has significantly negative coefficients for all dimensions ($p<0.01$). The interaction variable for smoking, excessive alcohol, and no exercises is negative and significant for the Mobility dimension, indicating an adverse synergetic health effect of bad health in several life-style factors, whereas the opposite is true for the Anxiety/depression scale.

Table 4 shows the contribution from each dimension to the concentration index according to Eq. 8 The predicted concentration index constitutes a large fraction of the observed concentration index leaving only a small fraction as the error residual. This is the case for the overall EQ-5D scores as well as the dimensions.

Table 3. Regression coefficients of EQ-5D and each of its dimensions ($n = 2915$)

	Mobility	Self-care	Usual activity	Pain/discomfort	Anxiety/depression	Dysfunctional	EQ-5D score
Ln(income)	0.0011	0.0001	0.0016*	0.0044*	0.0011	0.0040**	0.0123**
Male (31-45)	-0.0021	-0.0006	-0.0022	-0.0110**	-0.0032	-0.0154***	-0.0345***
Male (46-60)	-0.0033*	-0.0011	-0.0030	-0.0188***	-0.0036	-0.0161***	-0.0458***
Male (61-70)	0.0011	0.0015	0.0032	0.0007	0.0079	-0.0031	0.0113
Male (71-80)	0.0035	0.0016	0.0004	0.0012	0.0105*	-0.0089	0.0083
Female (16-30)	-0.0011	-0.0004	-0.0028	-0.0019	-0.0074**	-0.0148***	-0.0285**
Female (31-45)	-0.0011	-0.0009	-0.0032*	-0.0186***	-0.0075**	-0.0252***	-0.0566***
Female (46-60)	-0.0039*	-0.0027*	-0.0041**	-0.0182***	-0.0051	-0.0235***	-0.0574***
Female (61-70)	0.0058**	0.0039*	0.0005	-0.0097	-0.0040	-0.0166**	-0.0202
Female (71-80)	0.0038	-0.0043*	-0.0067**	-0.0029	0.0000	-0.0184**	-0.0285
Low Education	-0.0032*	-0.0014	-0.0018	-0.0048	-0.0031	-0.0038	-0.0180
Medium Education	-0.0015	-0.0005	-0.0021	-0.0018	-0.0013	-0.0051	-0.0123
Other Education	-0.0007	0.0020	-0.0022	-0.0001	-0.0090	-0.0051	-0.0152
Skilled worker	-0.0017	-0.0007	-0.0021	0.0022	0.0009	-0.0017	-0.0032
White-collar worker	-0.0020	-0.0008	0.0000	0.0054	-0.0014	0.0021	0.0033
Selfemployed	-0.0003	-0.0003	0.0018	0.0076	0.0000	0.0038	0.0126
Assisting spouse	-0.0010	0.0007	0.0034	0.0073	-0.0003	0.0030	0.0132
Housewife	-0.0066*	0.0000	-0.0053	-0.0062	-0.0154**	-0.0124	-0.0458*
Apprentice	-0.0019	-0.006**	-0.0016	-0.0053	0.0081	-0.0118	-0.0187
Student	-0.0015	-0.0029	0.0014	-0.0040	0.0061	0.0066	0.0056
Retired	-0.0151***	-0.0067***	-0.0109***	-0.0238***	-0.0105***	-0.0205***	-0.0876***
Unemployed	-0.0058*	-0.0034	-0.0115***	-0.0064	-0.0223***	-0.0063	-0.0557***
Other job	-0.0050**	-0.0020	-0.0020	-0.0100	-0.0135***	-0.0082	-0.0407***
Cohabitant	-0.0003	0.0003	0.0016	0.0020	0.0023	0.0030	0.0088
Separated	0.0033	-0.0093**	0.0009	-0.0122	-0.0533***	-0.0189	-0.0895**
Divorced	-0.0065*	0.0003	-0.0045**	0.0055	-0.0126***	-0.0036	-0.0213*
Widowed	0.0016	-0.0005	0.0022	0.0061	-0.0058	0.0024	0.0061
Alone	-0.0005	-0.0006	0.0023	0.0022	-0.0008	0.0008	0.0033
Other	-0.0005	0.0030	0.0093	-0.0151	-0.0078	-0.0438*	-0.0549
Daily smoker	-0.0001	0.0004	-0.0009	-0.0099***	-0.0053***	-0.0042*	-0.0200***
High alcohol	0.0009	0.0018	0.0023	-0.0035	-0.0021	-0.0038	-0.0044
Vegetables, cooked	-0.0012	-0.0005	-0.0011	-0.0057**	0.0010	0.0005	-0.0071
Vegetables, raw	0.0008	0.0003	0.0002	0.0033	0.0011	0.0057**	0.0114*
Fruit	0.0008	0.0008	0.0005	-0.0022	0.0001	0.0016	0.0015
No exercises	-0.0131***	-0.0034***	-0.0114***	-0.0333***	-0.0091***	-0.0174***	-0.0878***
Smoker and alcohol	-0.0008	-0.0008	-0.0038	0.0126	-0.0094*	-0.0019	-0.0041
smoke,alco,no exer.	-0.0113**	-0.0062*	0.0051	-0.0087	0.0244***	0.0023	0.0057

*$P<0.10$, **$P<0.05$, ***$P<0.01$

The contributions from the regressors through the dimensions are shown in percentages of the overall predicted concentration index in Table 5. The regressors contribute to the overall concentration index with various magnitudes and signs. The largest contributors are income and being retired. Also men aged 31-45 or 46-60 years are large contributors, however with negative signs. The educational regressors contribute to the overall inequality, especially the

Table 4. Decomposition of observed/predicted CI and error CG into the six dimensions

	Mobility	Self-care	Usual activity	Pain/dis-comfort	Anxiety/depress.	Dysfunc-tional	EQ-5D Score
Predicted CI	0.00113	0.00051	0.00140	0.00333	0.00158	0.00299	0.01094
Observed weighted CI	0.00126	0.00046	0.00159	0.00392	0.00195	0.00382	0.01301
Error CG	0.00013	-0.00005	0.00019	0.00059	0.00037	0.00084	0.00207

n = 2915

residual category of other types of education. Of the life style variables only a life style with no exercises contributes considerably to the concentration index. As for the observed concentration indices, the different health dimensions contribute to the overall inequality to varying degree. Pain/discomfort and Dysfunctional are the most important contributors.

Discussion

The present study adds to earlier findings in Lauridsen et al. [19] by decomposing EQ-5D scores and by applying a Danish case, while Lauridsen et al. [19] applied 15D values to Finnish data. EQ-5D values are less straightforward to decompose than 15D values as the Danish EQ-5D values, established by Wittrup-Jensen et al. [15], differ from 15D values particularly in two ways. First, EQ-5D defines health as an endowment of perfect health, depreciated by moderate or severe health problems, while 15D is obtained as a sum of 15 health dimension contributions. This implies that inequality of health according to EQ-5D is to be interpreted as a weighted sum of inequality in ill-health, rather than inequality in contributions to health, as it is the case for the 15D values. Second, the Danish TTO model includes an indicator for any dysfunctional state. This implies that the contributions from the remaining five dimensions have to be interpreted as partial contributions, controlled for the contribution from having any dysfunctional states. Some national TTO models also include a variable for having any dimension scored at the worst state (e.g. the British TTO model [15, 17]). If such a TTO model had been used, this characteristic could have been incorporated in the sixth dimension. Despite these differences in interpretation, the present study shows that it is possible to encompass the EQ-5D into a methodological frame similar to that applied to the 15D by Lauridsen et al.[19]

Earlier findings reported by Lauridsen et al. [19] are largely confirmed by this analysis. That is, health status is a diversified matter, and an overall HRQL index may be too crude to measure health status for specific purposes. Policies combating inequalities in health might not show any changes in the overall index if decreases in inequality in one type of health are offset by increases in another. Therefore, it is relevant to know the sources of health status and health inequality.

Table 5. Contribution from each regressor and dimension to CI of EQ-5D (in percent of predicted CI) ($n = 2915$)

	Mobility	Self-care	Usual activity	Pain/dis-comfort	Anxiety/depress.	Dysfunc-tional	EQ-5D score
ln(income)	4.72	0.45	6.42	17.98	4.66	16.41	50.63
Male (31-45)	-1.48	-0.41	-1.55	-7.67	-2.27	-10.74	-24.12
Male (46-60)	-2.06	-0.66	-1.85	-11.78	-2.29	-10.10	-28.74
Male (61-70)	-0.06	-0.08	-0.18	-0.04	-0.43	0.17	-0.62
Male (71-80)	-0.39	-0.18	-0.05	-0.14	-1.20	1.01	-0.94
Female (16-30)	0.58	0.24	1.52	1.01	3.93	7.91	15.19
Female (31-45)	-0.13	-0.11	-0.39	-2.25	-0.91	-3.06	-6.85
Female (46-60)	-0.10	-0.06	-0.10	-0.44	-0.12	-0.57	-1.39
Female (61-70)	-1.60	-1.07	-0.13	2.68	1.12	4.61	5.60
Female (71-80)	-0.74	0.84	1.31	0.57	0.00	3.57	5.55
Low Education	0.30	0.12	0.16	0.44	0.28	0.35	1.65
Medium Education	-0.74	-0.25	-1.02	-0.88	-0.63	-2.48	-6.00
Other Education	0.52	-1.44	1.64	0.08	6.57	3.70	11.07
Skilled worker	-0.63	-0.24	-0.78	0.80	0.31	-0.62	-1.17
White-collar worker	-2.06	-0.80	0.02	5.59	-1.50	2.21	3.46
Selfemployed	-0.07	-0.08	0.44	1.86	0.01	0.94	3.09
Assisting spouse	0.01	-0.01	-0.05	-0.10	0.00	-0.04	-0.18
Housewife	0.56	0.00	0.45	0.53	1.31	1.06	3.90
Apprentice	0.16	0.51	0.14	0.45	-0.69	1.00	1.58
Student	1.01	1.97	-0.94	2.70	-4.08	-4.44	-3.78
Retired	11.14	4.93	8.04	17.52	7.71	15.08	64.42
Unemployed	0.42	0.25	0.83	0.46	1.62	0.46	4.04
Other job	-0.26	-0.10	-0.11	-0.53	-0.71	-0.43	-2.14
Cohabitant	-0.03	0.03	0.16	0.21	0.24	0.31	0.91
Separated	0.02	-0.07	0.01	-0.09	-0.38	-0.13	-0.63
Divorced	-0.19	0.01	-0.13	0.16	-0.38	-0.11	-0.64
Widowed	-0.24	0.07	-0.34	-0.94	0.89	-0.37	-0.94
Alone	0.36	0.45	-1.60	-1.50	0.52	-0.53	-2.30
Other	0.00	0.00	-0.01	0.01	0.01	0.03	0.04
Daily smoker	0.01	-0.03	0.06	0.68	0.36	0.29	1.37
High alcohol	0.02	0.03	0.04	-0.06	-0.04	-0.07	-0.08
Vegetables, cooked	-0.07	-0.03	-0.06	-0.32	0.05	0.03	-0.39
Vegetables, raw	0.08	0.03	0.02	0.35	0.11	0.60	1.20
Fruit	-0.08	-0.08	-0.05	0.24	-0.01	-0.17	-0.16
No exercises	1.11	0.29	0.96	2.82	0.77	1.47	7.43
Smoker and alcohol	0.01	0.01	0.05	-0.17	0.13	0.03	0.06
smoke,alco,no exer.	0.24	0.13	-0.11	0.18	-0.51	-0.05	-0.12
Predicted CI	10.34	4.65	12.82	30.42	14.47	27.31	100.00

Furthermore, the same factors seem to contribute to overall income-related inequality in Finland and Denmark, as income and being retired are the most important contributing factors. Some discrepancies, however, are found. In contrast to the findings of Lauridsen et al. [19], where Usual activities were found to be the most contributing factor, closely followed by Mental health, the present study found that Pain/discomfort and Dysfunctional were the most important factors. Further, in the Finnish case income is not contributing to inequality to the same degree as in the Danish, as the concentration index for income is somewhat higher in the Danish data than in the Finnish, indicating that income inequality is larger in Denmark than in Finland. Next, the findings of Lauridsen et al. [19] that education plays a role for some of the dimensions and for the overall score is only marginally confirmed. Finally, Lauridsen et al. [19] reported that being retired contributed about twice as much as income, while the two contributions were found to be approximately equal for the present study. These differences may be attributed to national differences as well as differences between 15D and EQ-5D.

The present study further added to the investigation of Lauridsen et al. [19] by including life-style variables as regressors. It is well documented that smoking, alcohol habits, and diet and activity patterns have an important influence on health.[24-27] Smoking and especially a sedentary life-style were the most important life style factors in the health regression models and the largest contributors to inequality. Although life style behavior is sometimes rooted in firmly cemented cultural habits, the possibilities of health policy initiatives might still have better chances of altering life-style than socioeconomic and sociodemographic conditions. Interaction terms were included, as the influence of different life style factors may act synergistically.[25, 28] The interaction terms of smoking, alcohol and sedentary behavior did not play a major role in the health regression models. However, they did contribute to the overall inequality, indicating that overall health inequality is a complicated pattern of life-style aspects and other socio-economic and socio-demographic circumstances.

The decomposition approach has been applied in an unpublished study by Gundgaard et al. with the SF-36 summary scores for physical and mental health. The results from the present study appear to be rather robust, as the results in the unpublished study showed the same tendencies. The most central findings are that income-related inequality in health is related mainly to lack of participation in the labor market, to income and to age distribution. Other socioeconomic and demographic determinants as well as life style factors do have some importance, but to a lesser degree.

Conclusion

The dimensions contributing most to overall EQ-5D income-related health inequality are pain/discomfort and being dysfunctional. Contributions from socioeconomic and life-style variables vary considerably. The most important factors are lack of participation in the labor market, income, and the age distribution. Of the life-style variables only a life-style with no exercises contributes considerably to the inequality. This implies that policy initiatives aiming at reducing income related health inequality will be more successful if directed toward specific aspects of health or certain socio-economic characteristics and life style factors. The results are robust in the sense that similar patterns were found in previous studies using 15D scores on Finnish data and SF-36 scores on Danish data, although discrepancies are found in relation to the former, which may be attributed to national differences and to conceptual differences between the scoring systems.

References

1. The Copenhagen declaration on reducing social inequalities in health *Scand J Public Health* 2002;**Suppl 59**:78-79.

2. Dahlgren G, Whitehead M. Policies and strategies to promote equity in health. 1-50. 2000. Copenhagen, WHO Regional Office for Europe.

3. Stronks G, Gunning-Schepers LJ. Should equity in health be target number 1. *Eur J Public Health* 1993;**65**:153-65.

4. Humphries KH and van Doorslaer E. Income-related health inequality in Canada. *Soc Sci Med* 2000;**50**:663-71.

5. Kakwani N, Wagstaff A, van Doorslaer E. Socioeconomic Inequalities in Health: Measurement, Computation, and Statistical Inference. *J Econometrics* 1997;**77**:87-103.

6. van Doorslaer E, Koolman X. Explaining the differences in income-related health inequalities across European countries. *Health Econ* 2004;**13**:609-28.

7. van Doorslaer E, Koolman X, Jones AM. Explaining income-related inequalities in doctor utilisation in Europe. *Health Econ* 2004;**13**:629-47.

8. van Doorslaer E, Wagstaff A, Bleichrodt H, Calonge S, Gerdtham UG, Gerfin M, Geurts J, Gross L, Hakkinen U, Leu RE, O'Donnell O, Propper C, Puffer F, Rodriguez M, Sundberg G, Winkelhake O. Income-related inequalities in health: some international comparisons. *J Health Econ* 1997;**16**:93-112.

9. Clarke PM, Gerdtham UG, Connelly LB. A note on the decomposition of the health concentration index. *Health Econ* 2003;**12**:511-16.

10. Wagstaff A, van Doorslaer E, Watanabe N. On Decomposing the Causes of Health Sector Inequalities with an Application to

Malnutrition Inequalities in Vietnam. *J Econometrics* 2003;**112**:207-23.

11. Brooks R. EuroQol: the current state of play. *Health Policy* 1996;**37**:53-72.

12. Brooks R. Quality of life measures. *Crit Care Med* 1996;**24**:1769.

13. Greiner W, Weijnen T, Nieuwenhuizen M, Oppe S, Badia X, Busschbach J, Buxton M, Dolan P, Kind P, Krabbe P, Ohinmaa A, Parkin D, Roset M, Sintonen H, Tsuchiya A, de Charro F. A single European currency for EQ-5D health states. *Eur J Health Econ* 2003;**4**:222-31.

14. The EuroQol Group. EuroQol--a new facility for the measurement of health-related quality of life. *Health Policy* 1990;**16**:199-208.

15. Wittrup-Jensen KU, Lauridsen J, Gudex C, Brooks R, Pedersen KM (2001) Estimating Danish EuroQol tariffs using the time trade-off (TTO) and visual analogue scale (VS) methods. In Norinder AL, Pedersen KM, Roos P (eds) Preceedings of the 18th Plenary Meeting of the EuroQol Group, 6th – 7th September 2001, Copenhagen, Denmark, IHE – The Swedish Institute for Health Economics, Lund.

16. Dolan P. Modeling valuations for EuroQol health states. *Med Care* 1997;**35**:1095-108.

17. Dolan P, Gudex C. Time preference, duration and health state valuations. *Health Econ* 1995;**4**:289-99.

18. Greiner W, Claes C, Busschbach J, Graf von der Schulenburg J-M. Validating the EQ-5D with time trade off for the German population. *Eur J Health Econ* 2005;**6**:124-30.

19. Lauridsen J, Christiansen T, Gundgaard J, Häkkinen U, Sintonen H. Decomposition of socio-economic determination of income-related health inequality by health domains. *Health Econ* 2006 [in press].

20. Sintonen H. The 15D instrument of health-related quality of life: Properties and applications. *Ann Med* 2001;**33**: 328-36

21. Boyle MH and Torrance GW. Developing multiattribute health indexes. *Med Care* 1984;**22**:1045-57.

22. Gundgaard J, Sørensen J. Evaluering af Fyns Amts Forebyggelsesstrategi: Baseline survey om sundhedstilstand og adfærd omkring tobak, alkohol, kost og motion [Evaluation of the Prevention Strategy in Funen County: Baseline Survey on Behaviour with respct to Tobacco, Alcohol, Diet and Exercise]. 2002. Funen County, Odense.

23. Kjøller M, Rasmussen NK. Sundhed og sygelighed I Danmark 2000 .... & udviklingen siden 1987 [Danish Health and Morbidity Survey 2000 .... & trends since 1989]. 2002. National Institute of Public Health, Copenhagen.

24. Ferrucci L, Izmirlian G, Leveille S, Phillips CL, Corti MC, Brock DB, Guralnik JM. Smoking, physical activity, and active life expectancy. *Am J Epidemiol* 1999;**149**:645-53.

25. McGinnis JM, Foege WH. Actual causes of death in the United States. *JAMA* 1993;**270**:2207-12.

26. Oguma Y, Sesso HD, Paffenbarger RS Jr., Lee IM. Physical activity and all cause mortality in women: a review of the evidence. *Br J Sports Med* 2002;**36**:162-72.

27. Paffenbarger RS Jr., Hyde RT, Wing AL, Lee IM, Jung DL, Kampert JB. The association of changes in physical-activity level and other life style characteristics with mortality among men. *N Engl J Med* 1993;**328**:538-545.

28. Robertson A, Tirado C, Lobstein T, Jermini M, Knai C, Jensen JH, Ferro-Luzzi A, James WTP. Food and health in Europe: a new basis for action. 2004. WHO, Copenhagen.

Chapter 6

Decomposition of sources of income-related health inequality applied on SF-36 summary scores: a Danish health survey

Jens Gundgaard, Jørgen Lauridsen

Health and Quality of Life Outcomes 2006; 4:53

Abstract

Background: If the SF-36 summary scores are used as health status measures for the purpose of measuring health inequality it is relevant to be informed about the sources of the inequality in order to be able to target the specific aspects of health with the largest impact.

Methods: Data were from a Danish health survey on health status, health behaviour and socio-economic background. Decompositions of concentration indices were carried out to examine the sources of income-related inequality in physical and mental health, using the physical and mental health summary scores from SF-36.

Results: The analyses show how the different subscales from SF-36 and various explanatory variables contribute to overall inequality in physical and mental health. The decompositions contribute with information about the importance of the different aspects of health and off-setting effects that would otherwise be missed in the aggregate summary scores. However, the complicated scoring mechanism of the summary scores with negative coefficients makes it difficult to interpret the contributions and to draw policy implications.

Conclusion: Decomposition techniques provide insights to how subscales contribute to income-related inequality when SF-36 summary scores are used.

Background

Equality in health is among the main objectives of health policy in many countries.[1-3] The present study considers the SF-36 instrument which is frequently used in health assessments or in health surveys to monitor health outcome as health-related quality of life (HRQoL). SF-36 has become one of the most widely used measures of health status,[4,5] and has also been used in studies of health inequalities.[6-10] The SF-36 consists of 8 scales for different dimensions of health. The 8 scales can be summarised into two summary scores for physical and mental health, respectively. If the summary scores are used as health status measures for the purpose of measuring inequality indices, it is relevant to be informed about the sources of health and inequality in health in order to be able to target the specific aspects of health with the largest potential impacts. The objective of this paper is to apply decomposition techniques to the two summary scores from SF-36 when concentration indices are used as measures for income-related inequality in health.

The analyses of the study follow the lines of Clarke et al.,[11] Wagstaff et al. [12] and Lauridsen et al.[13] Clarke et al. [11] decompose a concentration index by dimension and subgroup separately. In Wagstaff et al. [12] a multivariate regression approach is used for a decomposition of background characteristics. The regression approach assists a decomposition of a single characteristic's impact on inequality in a health component into 1) its regressive impact on the variation in the health component, and 2) the impact due to income-related inequality in the characteristic itself. In Lauridsen et al. [13] the decomposition by dimension from Clarke et al. [11] is merged with the regression approach from Wagstaff et al. [12]. The concentration indices are each decomposed into the different dimensions of health summing up to the respective index and the effect on health from different socio-economic characteristics. Lauridsen et al. [13] apply the decomposition on 15D summary scores from a Finnish survey. The analysis shows that the different components of health contribute to health and inequality in health to varying degree, and that relationships to socio-economic and socio-demographic characteristics vary considerably.

To summarise, the present study adds to the literature by showing how to apply the methodology of Lauridsen et al. [13] to Physical Component Score (PCS) and Mental Component Score (MCS) values of the SF-36. The method reveals how the different HRQoL dimensions and background characteristics contribute to overall inequality in physical and mental health-related quality of life.

Methods

Study participants

Five thousand people living in Funen County, Denmark aged 16-80 were drawn from The Centralised Civil Register to participate in a health survey on health status, health behaviour and socio-economic background. The sample was stratified with respect to municipalities and the data have been weighted by the reciprocals of the selection probabilities (taking unit-nonresponse into account). The data were gathered in the period from October 2000 through April 2001. An external response rate of 68 percent was obtained.[14] A number of the respondents had to be excluded due to item-nonresponse, leaving a final working sample of 2,767, or 55 percent. Gundgaard et al. [14] performed a descriptive response/nonresponse analysis and found that the number of women and men are approximately equal in the working sample. The participants are on average slightly younger than the nonparticipants. Middle-aged are slightly more prone to participate than the younger or older groups.[14]

Income was defined as previous year's gross income (gross of tax and deductibles) and measured as a categorical variable with 17 categories. The respondents were ranked according to their income category taking the sample weights into account. Within the categories the respondents were ranked randomly.

Health status was measured using the PCS and the MCS from SF-36, respectively.[4,15-21] The PCS and MCS were each calculated by standardising each of the eight dimensions from the Danish SF-36, multiplying each dimension by its respective factor score coefficient, summing and standardising to the American norm of a mean of 50 and a standard deviation of 10 as recommended in Ware et al. [22] and Bjorner et al.[15]

Statistical analysis

Income-related inequality in health was measured by the concentration index. The concentration index is a generalised Gini coefficient and is a measure of how equal one variable (HRQoL) is distributed with respect to the ranking of another variable (income).[23-25] The concentration index ranges between -1 and 1, and if it is positive then good health is concentrated among the higher income groups and vice versa. The concentration index can be estimated by ordinary least squares (OLS) regression and approximate standard errors and t-statistics are easily obtained.[23]

Concentration indices were estimated for PCS and MCS respectively. To explain the sources of income-related inequality in health these two indices were decomposed into components from the different dimensions of SF-36 and from explanatory background variables. The decompositions into dimensions were carried out as expressing the concentration indices for PCS and MCS as a weighted sum of concentration indices for the dimensions with the relative share of the HRQoL as weights.[11] The decomposition into explanatory variables was carried out by a multivariate regression approach as in Wagstaff et al.,[12] where the concentration indices for PCS and MCS were expressed as weighted sums of the concentration indices for the explanatory variables with the health elasticities with respect to the explanatory variables as weights.[12] The two decomposition techniques were merged together as in Lauridsen et al.[13] The concentration indices were then each decomposed into the different dimensions of health summing up to the respective indices PCS and MCS and the effect on health from different socio-demographic, socio-economic, and life-style characteristics. The technical details of the decomposition can be found in the appendix.

Results

Table 1 shows descriptive statistics and concentration indices with t-statistics for each of the eight individual scales and the overall score for PCS and MCS, respectively. The overall PCS is 51.80 with a standard deviation of 7.92 indicating that physical health status is slightly better than the American norm of 50. Furthermore, the variation is also smaller as the American norm is a standard deviation of 10. The concentration index of physical health using PCS with respect to income is 0.013. However, the concentration indices of the different scales present a large variation. All indices are statistically significant. The largest contributors to the overall concentration index for PCS are Physical Functioning, Role-Physical, and Bodily Pain. The MCS of 56.08 is somewhat better than the American norm of 50. The differential is bigger than half the standard deviation of 10 which is often considered to be the minimally important difference in HRQoL studies.[26] The variation is also smaller than the American counterpart. The income-related inequality in mental health status is lower than that of physical health status, as the overall concentration index for MCS is 0.008. The largest contributors to the overall concentration index for MCS are Role-Emotional and Mental Health.

Table 2 shows the contribution from each subscale to the concentration index. The predicted concentration indices for PCS and MCS constitute 86.3 and 74.9 percent, respectively, of the observed concentration indices. The different subscales contribute according to the sign of their coefficient. This means that for most subscales the contributions to overall health point in opposite directions for PCS and MCS.

The contributions from the different explanatory variables are shown in Tables 3 and 4 for PCS and MCS, respectively. As the contributions are rather small in absolute numbers, the contributions are shown in percentages of the overall predicted concentration indices. The different regressors contribute to the overall concentration index with various magnitudes and signs. For PCS the largest contributors are income and being retired. Also, the male 31-45 and 46-60 states are large contributors, however with negative signs. Furthermore, the educational regressors seem to play a role in the contribution to the overall inequality. Of the lifestyle variables, only a lifestyle with no exercises has a considerable contribution to the concentration index. For MCS, the largest contributors are being retired, being a white-collar worker (diminishes the inequality), being a young female (aged 16-30), and income. Also for MCS, the variable for no exercises plays a role in explaining inequality in health.

Table 1. Descriptive statistics and concentration indices of PCS and MCS and each of its dimensions

	Mean	SD	C_i	t*	Weight	PCS Contr	PCS Contr (%)	Weight	MCS Contr	MCS Contr (%)
Physical Function (PF)	93.24	14.55	0.017	9.56	0.333	0.006	44.4	-0.167	-0.003	-36.6
Role-Physical (RP)	87.47	28.65	0.026	6.84	0.175	0.005	35.4	-0.057	-0.001	-18.9
Bodily Pain (BP)	83.18	24.42	0.019	5.37	0.216	0.004	31.4	-0.061	-0.001	-14.6
General Health Perception (GH)	75.63	15.39	0.015	6.16	0.181	0.003	21.1	-0.011	0.000	-2.0
Vitality Scale (VT)	74.40	20.23	0.019	6.10	0.020	0.000	2.9	0.150	0.003	36.0
Social Function (SF)	95.57	13.74	0.007	4.25	-0.006	0.000	-0.3	0.205	0.001	18.2
Role-Emotional (RE)	91.49	24.09	0.018	5.89	-0.103	-0.002	-14.0	0.214	0.004	48.2
Mental Health (MH)	86.88	15.29	0.013	6.55	-0.205	-0.003	-20.8	0.418	0.005	69.7
PCS	51.80	7.92	0.013	7.10	1.000	0.013	100.0			
MCS	56.08	8.12	0.008	4.73				1.000	0.008	100.0

N=2767; Contr - Contribution; PCS – Physical component score; MCS – Mental component score; *Heteroskedasticity-robust standard errors obtained to calculate t-statistics.

Table 2. Decompositions of PCS and MCS concentration indices into contributions from dimensions

		PF	RP	BP	GH	VT	SF	RE	MH	Sum
PCS	Predicted C	0.00522	0.00382	0.00319	0.00221	0.00028	-0.00004	-0.00141	-0.00220	0.01108
	Observed C	0.00570	0.00454	0.00403	0.00271	0.00037	-0.00004	-0.00180	-0.00267	0.01284
	Error CG	0.00048	0.00073	0.00084	0.00050	0.00009	-0.00001	-0.00039	-0.00048	0.00176
MCS	Predicted C	-0.00262	-0.00124	-0.00090	-0.00013	0.00211	0.00121	0.00294	0.00447	0.00585
	Observed C	-0.00286	-0.00147	-0.00114	-0.00016	0.00281	0.00142	0.00376	0.00544	0.00781
	Error CG	-0.00024	-0.00022	-0.00024	-0.00003	0.00070	0.00021	0.00082	0.00097	0.00196

N=2767; PCS – Physical component score; MCS – Mental component score; PF - Physical Function; RP - Role-Physical; BP - Bodily Pain; GH - General Health Perception; VT - Vitality Scale; SF - Social Function; RE - Role-Emotional; MH - Mental Health (N=2767).

Table 3. Contribution from each regressor and each dimension to C of PCS (in percent of predicted C)

	PF	RP	BP	GH	VT	SF	RE	MH	PCS
Ln(income)	25.07	8.62	22.81	14.17	1.58	-0.02	-6.62	-7.44	58.17
Male (31-45)	-3.21	-4.38	-9.16	-5.68	-0.53	0.04	0.72	3.63	-18.58
Male (46-60)	-7.62	-5.66	-7.98	-8.29	-0.19	0.02	1.23	0.09	-28.43
Male (61-70)	-0.44	-0.60	-0.58	-0.24	-0.08	0.01	0.16	0.51	-1.26
Male (71-80)	1.17	0.14	-0.53	-0.16	-0.12	0.01	0.66	1.05	2.23
Female (16-30)	-0.18	0.44	1.90	1.22	0.57	-0.07	-2.86	-4.49	-3.46
Female (31-45)	-0.72	-1.41	-2.64	-1.45	-0.27	0.02	0.44	1.55	-4.48
Female (46-60)	-0.11	-0.12	-0.19	-0.10	-0.01	0.00	0.01	0.07	-0.44
Female (61-70)	0.81	-0.60	-0.75	-0.54	-0.16	-0.01	-0.47	-0.16	-1.88
Female (71-80)	3.90	3.52	1.42	1.24	0.20	0.00	-0.17	-1.16	8.95
Low Education	0.17	0.10	0.15	-0.03	0.00	0.00	0.03	-0.01	0.41
Medium Education	-0.34	-1.12	-2.75	2.07	0.09	-0.01	-0.52	-1.45	-4.04
Other Education	2.07	9.92	7.32	2.12	0.01	-0.03	-1.62	-1.95	17.84
Skilled worker	-1.46	-1.84	-0.92	-0.43	-0.08	0.00	0.24	0.99	-3.49
White-collar worker	-3.87	-1.02	7.05	-1.00	-0.17	0.04	1.55	6.43	9.02
Selfemployed	-0.31	-0.23	0.96	-0.66	0.01	-0.01	-0.23	0.99	0.52
Assisting spouse	-0.04	0.18	0.05	0.04	0.01	0.00	-0.03	-0.05	0.16
Housewife	1.33	2.57	0.31	1.44	0.15	-0.03	-0.17	-2.00	3.60
Apprentice	0.59	0.28	0.70	-0.23	0.01	0.00	0.64	0.31	2.30
Student	0.83	-2.32	-2.50	-3.21	0.14	-0.03	2.14	-2.34	-7.28
Retired	28.02	24.08	15.63	18.38	1.18	-0.22	-5.73	-9.38	71.94
Unemployed	1.29	1.82	0.02	1.09	0.06	-0.03	-0.23	-1.17	2.84
Other job	-0.67	-0.78	-0.19	-0.43	-0.02	0.01	0.27	0.64	-1.17
Cohabitant	0.13	0.10	0.36	0.21	0.02	0.00	0.01	-0.09	0.74
Separated	-0.04	-0.12	-0.14	-0.01	-0.02	0.00	0.01	0.30	-0.02
Divorced	-0.56	-0.35	-0.07	-0.21	-0.04	0.01	0.25	0.34	-0.62
Widowed	0.15	-0.12	-0.35	-0.44	-0.02	-0.01	-1.31	-1.06	-3.15
Alone	-2.22	1.69	-3.06	-0.33	-0.06	0.00	-0.40	-2.60	-6.99
Other	0.02	0.03	-0.04	-0.06	0.00	0.00	-0.03	-0.01	-0.09
Daily smoker	0.13	0.29	0.56	0.39	0.05	-0.01	-0.11	-0.22	1.09
High alcohol	0.01	0.00	-0.15	-0.12	0.01	0.00	-0.06	-0.14	-0.46
Vegetables, cooked	-0.07	-0.39	-0.25	-0.08	0.02	0.00	-0.03	-0.12	-0.93
Vegetables, raw	0.24	0.03	0.16	0.29	0.07	0.00	0.01	-0.31	0.50
Fruit	0.09	-0.01	-0.13	0.03	0.00	0.00	-0.01	0.02	-0.02
No exercises	2.56	1.40	1.30	0.85	0.15	-0.02	-0.51	-0.71	5.03
Smoker and alcohol	0.02	-0.02	-0.01	0.01	0.01	0.00	-0.03	-0.09	-0.12
Smoke,alco,no exer	0.38	0.34	0.49	0.11	-0.03	0.00	0.07	0.20	1.57
Predicted C	47.11	34.46	28.80	19.95	2.52	-0.33	-12.70	-19.83	100.00

N=2767; PF - Physical Function; RP - Role-Physical; BP - Bodily Pain; GH - General Health Perception; VT - Vitality Scale; SF - Social Function; RE - Role-Emotional; MH - Mental Health.

Discussion

The study reproduced the methods of Lauridsen et al. [13] in order to carry out decompositions of health status measures using the PCS and the MCS from SF-36, while Lauridsen et al. [13] applied 15D as health status measure.

The findings in Lauridsen et al. [13] were confirmed herein. That is, health status is a diversified matter, and an overall index may be too crude to health status for specific purposes. Policies combating inequalities in health might not produce any changes in the overall index if decreases in inequality in one type of health are offset by increases in another. Therefore, it is important to know the sources of health status and health inequality. For the specific dimensions of health the policies can be directed towards the distribution of the explanatory variables, modifying the relationship between the explanatory variables and health (with, for example, more health care or preventive measures targeted specific groups), or redistributing income between groups. It is important to note that the distribution of some of the explanatory variables are not modifiable (e.g. age, gender), and the estimated health effects of some characteristics are not necessarily applicable to all groups (e.g. due to self-selection). Furthermore, the basis for policy is also restricted by normative considerations.

Compared to 15D, the summary scores from SF-36 were not as straightforward to decompose. A summary score from SF-36 is complicated as the score is a function of eight other scores each building on several items. In the present analysis the eight SF-36 scores were taken as given, and there were no focus on the original items. In principle, the decomposition could have been carried out on the original items. However, decomposing a summary score into the different items might not have contributed with more relevant information. The relevant choice of level of decomposition depends on the focus of the analysis.

To correct for the confounding of physical and mental health, negative coefficients for some subscales subtract back the unwanted variance. This scoring mechanism has caused some controversy as a maximum score of PCS is achieved only when the mental health scales are at a low level and vice versa for MCS.[19-21, 27] It is outside the scope of this article, however, to assess the scoring mechanism for the SF-36 summary scores. Nevertheless, the negative coefficients do make it harder to interpret the contributions to the decompositions as less inequality in some subscales tends to increase overall inequality. Furthermore, the negative coefficients result in contributions in opposite directions to the two summary scores. This means that policies combating inequalities in physical health, as measured by PCS, tend to worsen inequality in mental health, as measured by MCS, and vice versa.

Table 4. Contribution from each regressor and each dimension to C of MCS (in percent of predicted C)

	PF	RP	BP	GH	VT	SF	RE	MH	MCS
ln(income)	-23.81	-5.30	-12.24	-1.56	22.58	1.31	26.19	28.66	35.84
Male (31-45)	3.05	2.70	4.92	0.63	-7.61	-2.71	-2.87	-13.98	-15.88
Male (46-60)	7.24	3.48	4.28	0.91	-2.79	-1.14	-4.87	-0.33	6.79
Male (61-70)	0.42	0.37	0.31	0.03	-1.17	-0.51	-0.64	-1.96	-3.16
Male (71-80)	-1.11	-0.09	0.28	0.02	-1.75	-0.71	-2.62	-4.04	-10.02
Female (16-30)	0.17	-0.27	-1.02	-0.13	8.23	4.43	11.31	17.29	40.00
Female (31-45)	0.68	0.87	1.42	0.16	-3.83	-1.10	-1.76	-5.96	-9.52
Female (46-60)	0.10	0.07	0.10	0.01	-0.15	-0.05	-0.05	-0.27	-0.23
Female (61-70)	-0.77	0.37	0.40	0.06	-2.31	0.40	1.86	0.63	0.64
Female (71-80)	-3.71	-2.16	-0.76	-0.14	2.85	-0.16	0.69	4.47	1.08
Low Education	-0.16	-0.06	-0.08	0.00	0.04	0.07	-0.11	0.03	-0.27
Medium Education	0.33	0.69	1.47	-0.23	1.27	0.51	2.07	5.59	11.71
Other Education	-1.96	-6.10	-3.93	-0.23	0.15	2.01	6.41	7.51	3.86
Skilled worker	1.38	1.13	0.49	0.05	-1.17	-0.22	-0.96	-3.81	-3.11
White-collar worker	3.67	0.63	-3.78	0.11	-2.45	-2.49	-6.15	-24.79	-35.26
Selfemployed	0.29	0.14	-0.51	0.07	0.21	0.91	0.93	-3.82	-1.79
Assisting spouse	0.04	-0.11	-0.03	0.00	0.15	-0.03	0.14	0.18	0.33
Housewife	-1.27	-1.58	-0.16	-0.16	2.20	1.85	0.67	7.72	9.27
Apprentice	-0.56	-0.17	-0.38	0.03	0.17	-0.25	-2.51	-1.21	-4.88
Student	-0.79	1.43	1.34	0.35	2.03	1.74	-8.48	9.02	6.64
Retired	-26.60	-14.80	-8.38	-2.03	16.85	13.79	22.69	36.16	37.68
Unemployed	-1.22	-1.12	-0.01	-0.12	0.81	1.88	0.93	4.50	5.65
Other job	0.64	0.48	0.10	0.05	-0.31	-0.84	-1.07	-2.46	-3.41
Cohabitant	-0.12	-0.06	-0.19	-0.02	0.30	-0.06	-0.05	0.35	0.15
Separated	0.04	0.07	0.08	0.00	-0.33	-0.11	-0.04	-1.16	-1.46
Divorced	0.53	0.21	0.04	0.02	-0.58	-0.70	-0.99	-1.30	-2.77
Widowed	-0.14	0.08	0.19	0.05	-0.22	0.83	5.17	4.08	10.03
Alone	2.11	-1.04	1.64	0.04	-0.92	0.13	1.60	10.00	13.56
Other	-0.01	-0.02	0.02	0.01	0.05	0.05	0.11	0.04	0.24
Daily smoker	-0.12	-0.18	-0.30	-0.04	0.76	0.45	0.45	0.86	1.88
High alcohol	-0.01	0.00	0.08	0.01	0.11	0.14	0.24	0.56	1.13
Vegetables, cooked	0.07	0.24	0.13	0.01	0.27	0.14	0.11	0.45	1.43
Vegetables, raw	-0.23	-0.02	-0.08	-0.03	0.97	0.18	-0.06	1.18	1.90
Fruit	-0.08	0.00	0.07	0.00	-0.02	0.10	0.05	-0.08	0.04
No exercises	-2.43	-0.86	-0.70	-0.09	2.09	1.08	2.01	2.72	3.81
Smoker and alcohol	-0.02	0.01	0.00	0.00	0.10	0.15	0.11	0.36	0.72
Smoke,alco,no exer	-0.36	-0.21	-0.26	-0.01	-0.45	-0.29	-0.29	-0.77	-2.64
Predicted C	-44.74	-21.18	-15.45	-2.20	36.15	20.76	50.24	76.42	100.00

N=2767; PF - Physical Function; RP - Role-Physical; BP - Bodily Pain; GH - General Health Perception; VT - Vitality Scale; SF - Social Function; RE - Role-Emotional; MH - Mental Health.

Conclusions

Decompositions of concentration indices with respect to the PCS and the MCS from SF-36 were carried out. When using SF-36 summary scores as health status measures the decompositions can be useful to reveal how the different subscales contribute to overall inequality. Furthermore, the decompositions allowed for explanatory variables to explain the sources of inequality. It was shown that the impact of socio-economic and health life style variables varied considerably. Income, gender, age, and being retired were the most important variables in explaining income-related inequality in physical and mental health. The decompositions also showed how the different subscales contributed to the PCS and the MCS. The decompositions into subscales turned out to be problematic as the complicated scoring mechanism of the summary scores produced contributions to inequality with opposite signs than expected.

Competing interests

The study was carried out thanks to a research grant from The Health Insurance Foundation, Denmark (Sygekassernes Helsefond). The authors alone are responsible for the contents of the article. No financial or non-financial competing interests exist.

Authors' contributions

Both authors participated in the design of the study, performed the statistical analyses, interpreted the results, and drafted the manuscript. Both authors read and approved the final manuscript.

Appendix

Like most generic HRQoL measures each of the PCS and MCS is comprised of dimensions that represent different aspects of health.[28] Like several other indices the final health status measure is calculated as a sum of scores for each dimension, i.e. as $Y = \sum_{i=1}^{I} Y_i$, where Y_i is the contribution to overall health from dimension i. The PCS and MCS of the SF-36 fit into this frame, as each of them can be written as

$$Y_j = 50 + 10 Y_j^{(raw)} = 50 + 10 \sum_{i=1}^{8} a_{ji} Y_i^{(Z)}$$

$$= 50 + 10 \sum_{i=1}^{8} a_{ji} \frac{Y_i - b_i}{c_i} = (50 - 10 \sum_{i=1}^{8} \frac{a_{ji} b_i}{c_i}) + \sum_{i=1}^{8} \frac{10 a_{ji}}{c_i} Y_i, \quad j = \text{PCS, MCS} \quad (1)$$

$$= v_{j0} Y_0 + \sum_{i=1}^{8} v_{ji} Y_i = \sum_{i=0}^{8} v_{ji} Y_i$$

where $Y_0 = 1$ and $Y_1, \ldots, Y_8$ are the raw scores on the 8 items. The income-related inequality for each of the items is measured by the concentration index C_i. If Y_i can be explained linearly by K regressors through linear regression then the concentration index can be decomposed into contributions from the regressors as

$$C_i = \sum_{k=1}^{K} \frac{\delta_{ik}\mu_k}{\mu_i} C_k + \frac{2}{\mu_i n} \sum_{n=1}^{N} \varepsilon_{i(n)} R_{(n)} = \sum_{k=1}^{K} \eta_{ik} C_k + \frac{1}{\mu_i} CG_{\varepsilon_i}, \qquad (2)$$

where δ_{ik}, μ_k and C_k are the OLS-coefficient, mean and concentration index of the k'th regressor,[12] and CG_{ε_i}/μ_i is a residual component of the inequality that cannot be explained. Using that the concentration index of $v_{ji}Y_i$ is equal to the concentration index of Y_i and that the concentration index of Y_0 is equal to zero, the concentration index of Y_j can also be decomposed into a weighted average [11]:

$$C_j = \sum_{i=0}^{8} w_{ji} C_i = \sum_{i=1}^{8} w_{ji} C_i, \qquad (3)$$

where C_j is the concentration index for Y_j, C_i the concentration index for Y_i, and w_{ij} a weight attached to the i'th dimension, estimated as $w_{ji} = \frac{v_{ji}\mu_i}{\mu_j}$, with μ_j and μ_i being the means of Y_j and Y_i respectively. Combining (2) and (3), the decomposition of C_j follows as in Lauridsen et al.[13]

$$C_j = \sum_{i=1}^{8} w_{ji} C_i = \sum_{i=1}^{8} v_{ji} \frac{\mu_i}{\mu_j} \left[\sum_{k=1}^{K} \frac{\delta_{ik}\mu_k}{\mu_i} C_k + \frac{1}{\mu_i} CG_{\varepsilon_i} \right]$$

$$= \sum_{i=1}^{8} \sum_{k=1}^{K} \frac{v_{ji}\delta_{ik}\mu_k}{\mu_j} C_k + \sum_{j=1}^{J} \frac{v_{ji}}{\mu_j} CG_{\varepsilon_i} \qquad j = \text{PCS, MCS.} \quad (4)$$

As demonstrated by Lauridsen et al. [13], the contribution from the k'th regressor to C_j^{PRED} is then obtained as $\sum_{i=1}^{8} \frac{v_{ji}\delta_{ik}\mu_k}{\mu_j} C_k$, while the contribution from the i'th dimension is obtained as $\sum_{k=1}^{K} \frac{v_{ji}\delta_{ik}\mu_k}{\mu_j} C_k$.

References

1. The Copenhagen declaration on reducing social inequalities in health. *Scand J Public Health* 2002;**Suppl 59**:78-79.

2. Dahlgren G, Whitehead M. Policies and strategies to promote equity in health. Copenhagen: WHO Regional Office for Europe; 2000.

3. Stronks G, Gunning-Schepers LJ. Should equity in health be target number 1. *Eur J Public Health* 1993;**65**:153-65.

4. Brazier J. The SF-36 health survey questionnaire--a tool for economists. *Health Econ* 1993;**2**:213-15.

5. Yost KJ, Haan MN, Levine RA, Gold EB. Comparing SF-36 scores across three groups of women with different health profiles. *Qual Life Res* 2005;**14**:1251-61.

6. Lahelma E, Martikainen P, Rahkonen O, Roos E, Saastamoinen P. Occupational class inequalities across key domains of health: Results from the Helsinki Health Study. *Eur J Publ Health* 2005;**15**:504-10.

7. Skapinakis P, Lewis G, Araya R, Jones K, Williams G. Mental health inequalities in Wales, UK: multi-level investigation of the effect of area deprivation. *Br J Psychiatry* 2005;**186**:417-22.

8. Isacson D, Bingefors K, von Knorring L. The impact of depression is unevenly distributed in the population. *Eur Psychiatry* 2005;**20**:205-12.

9. Yamazaki S, Fukuhara S, Suzukamo Y. Household income is strongly associated with health-related quality of life among Japanese men but not women. *Public Health* 2005;**119**:561-67.

10. Clarke P, Smith L, Jenkinson C. Comparing health inequalities among men aged 18-65 years in Australia and England using SF-36. *Aust N Z J Public Health* 2002;**26**:136-143.

11. Clarke PM, Gerdtham UG, Connelly LB. A note on the decomposition of the health concentration index. *Health Econ* 2003;**12**:511-16.

12. Wagstaff A, van Doorslaer E, Watanabe N. On Decomposing the Causes of Health Sector Inequalities with an Application to Malnutrition Inequalities in Vietnam. *J Econometrics* 2003;**112**:207-223.

13. Lauridsen J, Christiansen T, Gundgaard J, Häkkinen U, Sintonen H. Decomposition of health inequality by determinants and dimensions. *Health Econ*, In press.

14. Gundgaard J, Sørensen J. [Evaluation of the Prevention Strategy in Funen County: Baseline Survey on Behaviour with respct to Tobacco, Alcohol, Diet and Exercise]. Funen County 2002.

15. Bjorner JB, Damsgaard MT, Watt T, Bech P, Rasmusen NK, Kristensen TS, Modvig J, Thunedborg K. Danish Manual for SF-36. Lif Lægemiddelindustriforeningen 1997.

16. Adler NE, Ostrove JM. Socioeconomic status and health: what we know and what we don't. *Ann N Y Acad Sci* 1999;**896**:3-15.

17. Bjorner JB, Thunedborg K, Kristensen TS, Modvig J, Bech P. The Danish SF-36 Health Survey: translation and preliminary validity studies. *J Clin Epidemiol* 1998;**51**:991-99.

18. Jenkinson C. The SF-36 physical and mental health summary measures: an example of how to interpret scores. *J Health Serv Res Policy* 1998;**3**:92-96.

19. Ware JE, Kosinski M. Interpreting SF-36 summary health measures: a response. *Qual Life Res* 2001;**10**:405-13.

20. Wilson D, Parsons J, Tucker G. The SF-36 summary scales: problems and solutions. *Soz Praventivmed* 2000;**45**:239-46.

21. Simon GE, Revicki DA, Grothaus L, Vonkorff M. SF-36 summary scores: are physical and mental health truly distinct? *Med Care* 1998;**36**:567-72.

22. Ware JE, Gandek B, Kosinski M, Aaronson NK, Apolone G, Brazier J, Bullinger M, Kaasa S, Leplège, Prieto L, Sullivan M, Thunedborg. The Equivalence of SF-36 Summary Health Scores Estimated Using Standard and Country-Specific Algorithms in 10 Countries: Results from the IQOLA Project. *J Clin Epidemiol* 1998;**51**:1167-70.

23. Kakwani N, Wagstaff A, van Doorslaer E. Socio inequalities in health: measurement, computation, and statistical inference. *J Econometrics* 1997;**77**:87-103.

24. van Doorslaer E, Wagstaff A, Bleichrodt H, Calonge S, Gerdtham UG, Gerfin M, Geurts J, Gross L, Häkkinen U, Leu RE, O'Donnell O, Propper C, Puffer F, Rodriguez M, Sundberg G, Winkelhake O. Income-related inequalities in health: some international comparisons. *J Health Econ* 1997;**16**:93-112.

25. Koolman X, van Doorslaer E. On the interpretation of a concentration index of inequality. *Health Econ* 2004;**13**:649-56.

26. Norman GR, Sloan JA, Wyrwich KW. Interpretation of Changes in Health-related Quality of Life: The Remarkable Universality of Half a Standard Deviation. *Med Care* 2003;**41**:582-92.

27. Taft C, Karlsson J, Sullivan M. Do SF-36 summary component scores accurately summarize subscale scores? *Qual Life Res* 2001;**10**:395-404.

28. Boyle MH, Torrance GW. Developing multiattribute health indexes. *Med Care* 1984;**22**:1045-57.

Chapter 7

The effect of non-response on estimates of health care utilization:

Linking health surveys and registers

Jens Gundgaard, Ola Ekholm,
Ebba Holme Hansen, Niels Kr. Rasmussen

European Journal of Public Health 2008; 18: 189-194

Abstract

Objective: Non-response in health surveys may lead to bias in estimates of health care utilization. The magnitude, direction and composition of the bias are usually not well known. When data from health surveys are merged with data from registers at the individual level, analyses can reveal non-response bias. Our aim was to estimate the composition, direction and magnitude of non-response bias in the estimation of health care costs in two types of health interview surveys.

Methods: The surveys were (1) a national personal interview survey of 22,484 Danes, (2) a telephone interview survey of 5,000 Danes living in Funen County. Data were linked with register information on health care utilization in hospitals and primary care. Health care utilization was estimated for respondents and non-respondents, and the difference was explained by a decomposition method of bias components.

Results: The surveys produced the same pattern of non-response, but with slight differences in non-response bias. Response rates for the interview and telephone surveys were 75% and 69%, respectively. Refusal was the most frequent reason for non-response (22% and 20% of those sampled, respectively), whereas illness, non-contact, and other reasons were less frequent. Respondents used 3% to 6% less health care than non-respondents at the aggregate level, but the opposite was true for some specific types of health care. Non-response due to illness was the main contributor to non-response bias.

Conclusion: Different types of non-response have different bias effects. Refusal is the most frequent reason for non-response, but illness is the most important contributor to non-response bias. The results encourage the continued use of interview health surveys.

Keywords: non-response, health care, utilization, health survey, registers, bias

Background

Health interview surveys contribute important information on health status, health behavior and health care utilization in the population. A health survey is often the only source of information when variables of interest are not available from registers. The problem with surveys is, of course, that not all the people who are invited to participate do so. Failure to participate can lead to bias in estimates on the population. If missing data are randomly unavailable for unknown reasons, the non-response might not interfere with the survey's intention to be representative. However, when non-response is systematically related to the variables of interest, the potential effect of non-response needs scrutiny.[1-3] This may well be the case for health surveys, as illness can be one of the reasons for not participating.[4-6] The bias of the non-response is determined by the multiplicative effect of the proportion of non-respondents and the difference between the respondents and non-respondents.[7] Furthermore, different types of non-response may have different or off-setting effects on the magnitude and direction of the bias.[7] The magnitude, direction and composition of the bias are usually not well known and the problem of non-response bias tends to be ignored. This is in keeping with the purpose of conducting a population survey, which is to collect information not available from other sources. Although the issue of non-response is as old as survey research itself, its importance does not appear to decrease.[8] Although not unequivocal, there are signs that it is increasingly difficult to obtain high response rates.[7-9] The climate for taking surveys may deteriorate due to societal changes such as increased urbanization and changing demographic and family structures, and decreasing norms for civic duty.[7] In addition, over-surveying in some countries and public debates on invasion of privacy and confidentiality may worsen conditions even more.[7,8]

There is no general agreement about which mode of interview (face-to-face or telephone) results in the highest response rates, and both have been mentioned.[10,11] The two modes are not usually directly comparable, as different design features are applied, in addition to the mode of interview.

Previous studies support the presumption that non-response is a complex phenomenon made up of various effects, especially when the focus is on health care utilization. Concerning hospital admissions, some studies showed higher utilization among non-respondents,[12-17] while other studies showed no differences between respondents and non-respondents.[4,18-20] A Danish study showed that the non-respondents in general had the same admission rates as the respondents, but the admission rates were higher among non-respondents around the interview period. The pattern is even more diverse for primary health care. Some studies registered lower health care utilization for non-respondents,[4,18,19] whereas other studies showed higher health care utilization rates.[21,22]

The present study focuses on the representativeness of estimates of health care utilization among respondents in sampled surveys by obtaining information on health care utilization from registers for respondents as well as non-respondents. The aim of the article is twofold: 1) to estimate the magnitude, direction and composition of non-response bias in health care utilization, and 2) to compare the non-response bias from two sources of health surveys: a personal interview survey and a telephone interview survey.

Methods

Personal interview data

The personal interview data were obtained from The Danish Health Interview Survey 2000 (DHIS).[23,24] 22,484 Danish citizens aged 16 and above were drawn from the Centralized Civil Register to participate in a national health survey on health care utilization, health status, morbidity, health behavior, environmental and occupational health risks and health resources. The sample was stratified to include at least 1,000 respondents from each of the 15 Danish counties, and data were weighted by the reciprocals of the sampling probabilities. Data were collected from personal interviews by trained interviewers in three rounds in February, May, and September 2000, respectively. 16,688 individuals participated, corresponding to a weighted response rate of 74.5%.

Telephone interview data

The telephone interview data were obtained from The Funen County Health Survey (FCHS). Five thousand people living in Funen County, Denmark aged 16-80 were drawn from the Centralized Civil Register to participate in a health survey on health status, health behavior and socio-economic background. The sample was stratified with respect to municipalities, and the data were weighted by the reciprocals of the sampling probabilities. Data were gathered through telephone interviews from October 2000 through April 2001.[25] A total of 3,421 individuals participated, corresponding to a weighted response rate of 69.2%

Register-based data

Data from each survey were merged with data from individual-level computerized registers including: all somatic hospital visits, services in the primary health care sector such as GP visits, physiotherapy, specialist treatment, dentistry, and dispensed prescription medicine in 2000 and 2001. The use of registers to extract information on health care utilization makes it possible to obtain exact information on health care services over a long period of time. The registers also make it possible to distinguish between different types of health care, and the different types of services can be added by measuring health care utilization in monetary terms. Health care services were measured as the long-run costs of the services and approximated by prices, charges or fees.

Hospital visits were extracted from the National Patient Register and the Funen County Patient Administrative System (FPAS) and linked to DHIS and FCHS, respectively. These registers include records on somatic inpatient stays, ambulatory and emergency room visits. Each hospital admission was described by an estimated charge based on the 2002 Danish case-mix system of Diagnosis Related Groups (DRGs). The case-mix system covers inpatient hospital stays, whereas ambulatory and emergency room visits are described by a similar but simpler system. Capital costs are not included in the case-mix system. All charges were adjusted to 2003 price level for hospital treatments.[26]

The services in the primary health care sector were extracted from the Registry of Public Health Insurance and linked to DHIS and FCHS. This registry includes all partly or fully reimbursed health services in primary health care, i.e. from general practitioners, physiotherapists, dentists and specialists. Each service is described with a reimbursement fee. As considerable co-payment exists for dental health care and physiotherapy, these fees were adjusted to reflect the full amount (reimbursement + co-payment). Expert judgments were used to adjust the dental care fees to the approximate average level of dental care fees, whereas the relevant fees for physiotherapy where adjusted by dividing the reimbursement fees by the proportion of reimbursement. General practitioners are partly financed through capitation (about one-third of GP revenue), and the GP reimbursement fees were scaled up by this amount. All reimbursement fees were adjusted for inflation up to 2003 by the price index for physicians and physiotherapists.[26]

Medicine data were extracted from the Register of Medicinal Product Statistics (RMPS) and Odense University Pharmaco-epidemiologic Database (OPED) and linked to DHIS and FCHS, respectively.[27] These databases consist of all prescription refunds from Denmark and Funen County, respectively. The dispensed medicine is described by the total purchase price in the RMPS, whereas pharmacy retail prices including VAT are used for the OPED. A further difference is that OPED includes prescription medicine entitled to reimbursement, whereas RMPS includes all prescribed medicines. Neither of the databases contains information on over-the-counter-medicine. Medicines dispensed in hospitals are included in the hospital charges. The medicine prices were adjusted for inflation to the 2003 level by the index for pharmaceutical products and equipment.[26]

Statistical analyses

As non-response can have many causes, non-respondents were classified into different types of non-response along the lines of Kjøller and Thoning.[9] The following categories were used: *Interviewed, Refusals, Illness, Non-contacts*, and a residual category of *Other* (table 1). The category of interviewed consisted of partially or completely interviewed respondents. That is, the item non-response is included in the category of interviewed, as can be seen in the table. People living outside Funen County or registered as dead were regarded as not belonging to the parent population under investigation and were excluded from the full sample.[28]

Differences in health care utilization between respondents and non-respondents were analyzed with ANOVA. The effect of different types of non-response bias on the estimates of health care utilization has been analyzed in a decomposition framework. Groves and Couper suggest a decomposition of the survey estimate into components of bias from the different types of non-response:[7]

$$\mu_{interviewed} = \mu_n + \frac{m_{refusals}}{n}\left(\mu_{interviewed} - \mu_{refusals}\right) + \frac{m_{illness}}{n}\left(\mu_{interviewed} - \mu_{illness}\right) + \frac{m_{non-contacts}}{n}\left(\mu_{interviewed} - \mu_{non-contacts}\right) + \frac{m_{other}}{n}\left(\mu_{interviewed} - \mu_{other}\right), \quad (1)$$

where μ_j is the mean health care utilization for the different categories of non-response, m_j is the weighted number of people in the jth non-response category, and n is the weighted sample size. This formula makes it possible to quantify the effect on bias from the proportion of (the specific type of) non-respondents and the difference between the respondents and (the specific type of) non-respondents. Each of the differences in means was tested by a t-test for comparing two means.

Results

Table 1 displays the categorization of respondents and non-respondents for the two sources. The response rate was higher for the personal interview survey (74.5%) than the telephone survey (69.2%). The most frequent reason for non-response was refusal (22.1% and 20.3%, respectively). The non-contacts constituted the second largest category, which was larger in the telephone survey than in the interview survey (8% vs. 2%). Illness and hospital visits played a relatively minor role in the magnitude of non-response, although some refusals may have been due to health-related disabilities.

The mean health care costs for respondents and non-respondents are shown in table 2. The first column shows the mean health care costs for the overall representative samples for all sampled individuals. The figures are remarkably similar for both the interview and telephone surveys.

Table 1. Classification of respondents and non-respondents

	Interview survey (n=22 484)			Telephone survey (n=4985)[a]		
	n	n (wgt)[b]	%[b]	n	n (wgt)[b]	%[b]
Respondents						
Interviewed	16 688	16 741.6	74.5	3421	3449.8	69.2
Non-respondents						
Refusals						
Refusals	4755	4704.7	20.9	995	943.1	18.9
Refusals and cannot be contacted again	287	262.2	1.2	53	62.9	1.3
Illness/disabled						
Illness	87	88.9	0.4	37	34.9	0.7
Disabled	211	209.6	0.9	29	21.2	0.4
Non-contacts						
Gone away/hospital	51	55.0	0.2	56	52.0	1.0
Not contacted	263	273.6	1.2	273	280.3	5.6
Moved	56	60.3	0.3	49	52.1	1.1
No telephone				12	15.9	0.3
Other						
Other, including language problems	86	89.5	0.4	60	72.9	1.5

[a] Fifteen persons were excluded from the analysis due to oversampling (dead, moved outside Funen County).
[b] Data weighted by the reciprocals of the sampling probability.

The resulting non-response bias could be derived by comparing the first and second columns. Health care costs were a bit smaller for respondents at the overall level (DHIS: DKK 19,966; FCHS: DKK 19,073) than for the whole sampled population (DHIS: DKK 20,510; FCHS: DKK 20,254) (1 USD = 8.33 DKK, 2005 PPP),[29] An F-test for the differences between the respondents and non-respondents was only significant at a 10% level in the FCHS (F-statistics unavailable in the DHIS at the aggregate level). The interviewed had a significantly lower level of hospital utilization and medicines, and a higher level of dentistry in DHIS. In the telephone survey, which is a smaller sample, the interviewed had a lower level of hospital utilization and medicine use, and a higher level of specialist care and dentistry at a 10% level of significance.

The magnitude and composition of the non-response bias in health care utilization is illustrated in table 3 by applying Groves and Couper's decomposition.[7] The size of non-response bias for each type of health care consists of the proportion of the specific type of non-respondents (which is constant with respect to health care) and the difference between the interviewed and the specific type of non-respondents. The biggest contributor to non-response bias was illness. Although the ill or disabled constituted only about 1%, the large differential in health care utilization between the interviewed and the ill or disabled contributed to a considerable non-response bias component for the aggregate level (DHIS: DKK -615; FCHS: DKK -608). Refusal was the dominating reason for non-response, but the effect on non-response bias was not large, as the differential between the interviewed and those who refused was small.

Table 2. Mean health care costs 2000-2001 for respondents and non-respondents[a,b]

	All	Respondents	Non-respondents	F-value[c]	P-value
Interview survey (n=22 484)					
Hospital	12 285	11 844	13 571	4.90	0.0268
GP	1864	1848	1911	2.45	0.1177
Physiotherapy	436	435	438	0.01	0.9383
Specialist	692	684	717	1.47	0.2257
Dentist	1652	1727	1433	124.07	<0.0001
Medicine	3581	3428	4026	16.11	<0.0001
Total[d]	20 510	19 966	22 096	-	-
Telephone survey (n=4985)					
Hospital	13 304	12 203	15 778	3.08	0.0793
GP	1747	1711	1827	2.36	0.1246
Physiotherapy	367	391	314	1.24	0.2653
Specialist	573	606	499	4.33	0.0375
Dentist	1575	1654	1399	23.91	<0.0001
Medicine	2688	2509	3089	3.84	0.0500
Total	20 254	19 073	22 906	3.16	0.0755

[a] Both years included, Danish Kroner, 2003 price level (1 USD = 8.33 DKK, 2005 PPP).
[b] Data weighted by the reciprocals of the sampling probability.
[c] F-tests from ANOVA for H_0: $\mu_{respondents}=\mu_{non-respondents}$, based on stratification adjusted standard errors.
[d] F-test for aggregate health care costs not available as specific costs obtained from different servers.

At the aggregate level, all bias components were negative for the telephone survey, indicating that all types of non-response led to an underestimation of the magnitude of health care utilization. For the interview survey, the bias components were positive except for illness. The picture was less clear for the specific types of health care, and there was bias in different directions. The absolute sizes were rather small, although significant in some cases.

Discussion

The main findings of this study were that refusal was the most frequent reason for non-response, but that illness was the most important contributor to non-response bias. However, the non-response bias was small and insignificant in most cases. At the aggregate level, respondents used slightly less health care than the full sample. For some specific types of health care, typically in primary health care, the opposite was true. The analyses showed that non-response is a diversified matter. Different types of non-response have varied effects on the non-response bias. The ill/disabled constitute a small group among non-responders, but nevertheless consume a much higher level of health care than the interviewed. This should be expected, as health care utilization is directly influenced by this reason for non-response. This group of people may not be able to participate because they are too ill, i.e. the same reason that they need health care. Therefore, this pattern is most pronounced for types of health care such as hospitalization, GP visits and prescription medicine. The two modes of interview produced almost the same pattern of non-response, although the proportion of respondents was higher in the interview survey. However, some bias components had opposite effects in the two modes of interview.

Although the present study is not directly comparable with most of the studies in the literature, the results are in accordance with the main tendencies from previous findings: that hospital utilization is higher among non-respondents or that there are no differences between respondents and non-respondents.[4,12-20] As for the primary care utilization, the less clear pattern is also in accordance with the literature, with some studies showing lower and some studies higher health care utilization for non-respondents.[4,18,19,21,22]

Specific strengths of this study were that it used representative data from the general population and not only from a patient group or an insurance group, and investigated two modes of interview data. Linkage to registers made it possible to extract exact information on several types of health care in primary and secondary health care sectors for a long period of time. It also made it possible to measure health care utilization in monetary terms by applying fees and charges as proxies for the costs of the services. The advantage of using a common unit of measurement is that different types of health care services can be aggregated. Furthermore, the cost of the service reflects the complexity of the procedure. A visit to the doctor is not just a visit. A surgical procedure is quite different from a check-up, for example, and this would not have been reflected in health care measured by the number of visits or by a dichotomized variable for use/no-use, which is the normal unit of measurement in many health surveys. Furthermore, several services are often provided during one visit. Hence the number of visits, or a dichotomized variable for health care utilization, would not reflect the number of health care services.

Our study also has some limitations: although the analyses cover health care services from the primary care sector and hospital sector, some types of health care are not included in the analyses. For example, mental health care was not included with respect to hospital treatment. Furthermore, only services subject to partial or complete reimbursement by the Public Health Insurance system were included in the analyses. Private for-profit supply of some health care services does exist in Denmark, but plays a marginal although increasing role (for example, less than one percent of hospital beds are private). For dentistry, however, a considerable share of services is not reimbursed at all, and these services are not included in the registers. For medicine, only prescription medicine in the primary health care sector is in the database at the individual level (and in FCHS, only prescription medicine entitled to reimbursement and bought from pharmacies in Funen County). In addition, medicine used in hospitals, and medicine purchased illegally over the internet is not covered by the database (medicine used in hospitals is included in hospital charges). Furthermore, even though the two sources of data are sampled from general population groups, the FCHS is only a sample from one Danish county, whereas DHIS covers all of Denmark (although the county of Funen is generally supposed to be representative of the Danish population).[23,30] Some of the differences could be explained by regional differences.

Socio-demographic and socio-economic background characteristics are appropriate for providing a deeper understanding of non-response-bias. The relevant explanatory variables and appropriate statistical specifications could be further decomposed into bias components due to socio-demographic/economic differences across non-response groups and components due to different utilization patterns across non-response groups. This would give new insight into the composition of non-response bias.

Table 3. Mean health care costs 2000-2001[a] and proportions of non-response: Estimation of the decomposition by bias component

	Interviewed	All		Refusals[b,c]		Illness[b,c]		Non contacts[b,c]		Other[b,c]	
	μ_{int}	=	μ_n	$+ (m_{ref}/n)*(\mu_{int}-\mu_{ref})$		$+ (m_{ill}/n)*(\mu_{int}-\mu_{ill})$		$+ (m_{nc}/n)*(\mu_{int}-\mu_{nc})$		$+ (m_o/n)*(\mu_{int}-\mu_o)$	
Interview survey (n=22 484)[d]											
All components											
Hospital	11 844	12 285		0.22	110	0.01	-35 093**	0.02	-31	0.00	274
GP	1848	1864		0.22	18	0.01	-1605**	0.02	164	0.00	-373
Physiotherapy	435	436		0.22	53	0.01	-1194**	0.02	227*	0.00	-126
Specialist	684	692		0.22	-62*	0.01	189*	0.02	110	0.00	183
Dentist	1727	1652		0.22	229**	0.01	865**	0.02	600**	0.00	695**
Medicine	3428	3581		0.22	-191	0.01	-9390**	0.02	743*	0.00	282
Total[e]	19 966	20 510		0.22	157	0.01	-46 228	0.02	1813	0.00	935
– *Size of bias*											
Hospital	11 844	12 285			24		-467		-1		1
GP	1848	1864			4		-21		3		-1
Physiotherapy	435	436			12		-16		4		-1
Specialist	684	692			-14		3		2		1
Dentist	1727	1652			51		12		10		3
Medicine	3428	3581			-42		-125		13		1
Total	19 966	20 510			35		-615		31		4

[a] Both years included, Danish Kroner, 2003 price level (1 USD = 8.33 DKK, 2005 PPP).
[b] The proportion of non-response for type j (m_j/n) remains constant for all types of health care.
[c] T-tests for H_0: ($\mu_{int}-\mu_j$)=0, based on stratification adjusted standard errors, *p<0.05, **p<0.01.
[d] Data weighted by the reciprocals of the sampling probability.
[e] T-tests for aggregate health care costs not available as specific costs have been obtained from different servers.

Table 3. (Continued)

	Interviewed	All	Refusals[b,c]		Illness[b,c]		Non contacts[b,c]		Other[b,c]	
Telephone survey (n=4985)[d]										
All components										
Hospital	12 203	13 304	0.20	-974	0.01	-41 902**	0.08	-3480	0.01	-10 504
GP	1711	1747	0.20	56	0.01	-1967**	0.08	-210	0.01	-549
Physiotherapy	391	367	0.20	130*	0.01	-1543	0.08	130	0.01	281**
Specialist	606	573	0.20	92	0.01	192	0.08	93	0.01	323**
Dentist	1654	1575	0.20	137*	0.01	883**	0.08	440**	0.01	385**
Medicine	2509	2688	0.20	-300	0.01	-9685**	0.08	-85	0.01	-170
Total	19 073	20 254	0.20	-858	0.01	-54 023**	0.08	-3111	0.01	-10 235
Size of bias										
Hospital	12 203	13 304		-197		-471		-279		-154
GP	1711	1747		11		-22		-17		-8
Physiotherapy	391	367		26		-17		10		4
Specialist	606	573		19		2		7		5
Dentist	1654	1575		28		10		35		6
Medicine	2509	2688		-60		-109		-7		-2
Total	19 073	20 254		-173		-608		-250		-150

[a] Both years included, Danish Kroner, 2003 price level (1 USD = 8.33 DKK, 2005 PPP).
[b] The proportion of non-response for type j (m_j/n) remains constant for all types of health care.
[c] T-tests for H_0: ($\mu_{int}-\mu_j$)=0, based on stratification adjusted standard errors, *p<0.05, **p<0.01.
[d] Data weighted by the reciprocals of the sampling probability.
[e] T-tests for aggregate health care costs not available as specific costs have been obtained from different servers.

Conclusion

The two modes of interview (personal and telephone) produce the same pattern of non-response, but do not produce the same non-response bias with respect to health care utilization. Refusal is the most frequent reason for non-response, whereas illness is the most important contributor to non-response bias.

There seems to be a trend towards decreasing participation rates in health interview surveys. However, the general validity of the results may not be threatened by the bias produced by non-response, although the underreporting caused by non-participating ill people is an important component that should be taken into consideration in surveys based on general populations.

Acknowledgements

The authors would like to thank Funen County and OPED for supplying data for the analyses of the Funen population. The Funen County Health Survey was partly funded by a research grant from The Health Insurance Foundation, Denmark (Sygekassernes Helsefond). The National Health Interview Survey was funded by the National Institute of Public Health and The Ministry of Interior and Health. The authors alone are responsible for the contents of the article.

References

1. Greene WH. *Econometric Analysis*. 4 ed.Prentice Hall, 2000.

2. Perneger TV, Chamot E, Bovier PA. Nonresponse bias in a survey of patient perceptions of hospital care. *Med Care* 2005;**43**:374-80.

3. Cohen G, Duffy JC. Are Nonrespondents to Health Surveys Less Healthy Than Respondents. *J Official Statistics* 2002;**18**:13-23.

4. Lamers LM. Medical consumption of respondents and non-respondents to a mailed health survey. *Eur J Public Health* 1997;**7**:267-71.

5. Boersma F, Eefsting JA, van den Brink W, van Tilburg W. Characteristics of non-responders and the impact of non-response on prevalence estimates of dementia. *Int J Epidemiol.* 1997;**26**:1055-62.

6. Macera CA, Jackson KL, Davis DR, Kronenfeld JJ, Blair SN. Patterns of non-response to a mail survey. *J Clin Epidemiol* 1990;**43**:1427-30.

7. Groves RM, Couper MP. Nonresponse in Household Interview Surveys.Wiley Interscience, 1998.

8. de Heer W. International Response Trends: Results of an International Survey. *J Official Statistics* 1999;**15**:129-42.

9. Kjoller M, Thoning H. Characteristics of non-response in the Danish Health Interview Surveys, 1987-1994. *Eur J Public Health* 2005;**15**:528-35.

10. Bowling B. *Research Methods in Health: Investigating Health and Health Services*. 2 ed. Buckingham, Philadelphia: Open University Press, 2002.

11. Frankfort-Nachmias C, Nachmias D. *Research Methods in the Social Sciences*. 5 ed. London: Arnold, 1996.

12. Osler M, Schroll M. Differences Between Participants and Nonparticipants in A Population Study on Nutrition and Health in the Elderly. *Eur J Clin Nutr* 1992;**46**:289-95.

13. Vestbo J, Rasmussen FV. Baseline characteristics are not sufficient indicators of non-response bias follow up studies. *J Epidemiol Community Health* 1992;**46**:617-19.

14. Paganini-hill A, Hsu G, Chao A, Ross RK. Comparison of Early and Late Respondents to A Postal Health Survey Questionnaire. *Epidemiology* 1993;**4**:375-79.

15. Jackson R, Chambless LE, Yang K, Byrne T, Watson R, Folsom A, Shahar E, Kalsbeek W. Differences between respondents and nonrespondents in a multicenter community-based study vary by gender ethnicity. The Atherosclerosis Risk in Communities (ARIC) Study Investigators. *J Clin Epidemiol* 1996;**49**:1441-46.

16. Janzon L, Hanson BS, Isacsson SO, Lindell SE, Steen B. Factors influencing participation in health surveys. Results from prospective population study 'Men born in 1914' in Malmo, Sweden. *J Epidemiol Community Health* 1986;**40**:174-77.

17. Drivsholm T, Eplov LF, Davidsen M et al. Representativeness in population-based studies: A detailed description of non-response in a Danish cohort study. *Scand J Public Health* 2006;**34**:623-31.

18. Reijneveld SA, Stronks K. The impact of response bias on estimates of health care utilization in a metropolitan area: the use of administrative data. *Int J Epidemiology* 1999;**28**:1134-40.

19. Etter JF, Perneger TV. Analysis of non-response bias in a mailed health survey. *J Clin Epidemiol* 1997;**50**:1123-28.

20. Rupp I, Triemstra M, Boshuizen HC, Jacobi CE, Dinant HJ, van den Bos GA. Selection bias due to non-response in a health survey among patients with rheumatoid arthritis. *Eur J Public Health* 2002;**12**:131-35.

21. Grotzinger KM, Stuart BC, Ahern F. Assessment and control of nonresponse bias in a survey of medicine use by the elderly. *Med Care* 1994;**32**:989-1003.

22. Korkeila K, Suominen S, Ahvenainen J et al. Non-response and related factors in a nation-wide health survey. *Eur J Epidemiol* 2001;**17**:991-99.

23. Kjøller M, Rasmussen NK. *Danish Health and Morbidity Survey 2000 ... & trends since 1989* (in Danish). National Institute of Public Health. 2002.

24. Davidsen M, Kjøller M. The Danish Health and Morbidity Survey 2000 - Design and Analysis. *Statistics in Transition* 2002;**5**:927-42.

25. Gundgaard J, Sørensen J. *Evaluation of the Prevention Strategy in Funen County: Baseline Survey on Behaviour with respct to Tobacco, Alcohol, Diet and Exercise* (in Danish). Funen County. 2002.

26. Statistics Denmark. StatBank Denmark, PRIS6. www.dst.dk . (28-10-2003).

27. Hallas J. Conducting pharmacoepidemiologic research in Denmark. *Pharmacoepidemiol Drug Saf* 2001;**10**:619-23.

28. Section for Survey Statistics and Swedish Statistician Society. Standard for Non-response Calculations. 2005.

29. OECD. *Purchasing Power Parities - Comparative Price Levels*. Main Economic Indicators. 2006.

30. Bjerrum L, Søgaard J, Hallas J, Kragstrup J. Polypharmacy in general practice: differences between practitioners. *Br J Gen Pract* 1999;**49**:195-98.

Chapter 8

Discussion

Contents of Chapter 8

DISCUSSION	**235**
Summing up	**235**
Research contribution	235
Overall results	236
Policy implications	237
Limitations	**241**
Focus of the study	241
Assumptions	242
The cross-sectional design	243
The health care variable	244
The health variable	245
The income variable	248
Econometric specifications	249
Generalizability	250
Future research	**252**
CONCLUSION	**256**
REFERENCES	**259**

Discussion

Summing up

Research contribution

The thesis adds to existing knowledge in several ways. It has utilized the combination of a health survey and registers to build a database with the relevant variables to carry out analyses on the distribution of health and health care in a geographical unit in Denmark. The database made it possible to use concentration indices to analyze the distribution of health by using two different HRQoL instruments (EQ-5D and SF-36), and to analyze the distribution of health care in monetary terms for six types of health care (hospital contacts, services at the GP, physiotherapist, specialist, dentist, and prescription medicine) and health care at the aggregate level.

By using decomposition techniques the overall inequality measures have been decomposed into contributions from dimensions and determinants. For health the dimensions consisted of different aspects of health (subdimensions from the HRQoL instruments) and for health care the dimensions consisted of different types of health care. The determinants consisted of socio-demographic variables, socio-economic variables, and health-related life-style variables.

The thesis evaluates the Funen County health care system with respect to two principles: *equality in health* and *equal treatment for equal need* in the period around 2000 and 2001. As Funen was an integrated part of the Danish health care system at the time of data collection the study can also be perceived as a case study in the evaluation of the Danish health care system. The study contributes with policy relevant information per se. However, it can also be seen as the first point estimate in comparisons over time or as a validation of findings from international country comparisons.

Overall results

The analyses showed that good health is concentrated among the higher income groups. The concentration index has been estimated to 0.013 when EQ-5D TTO-values are used as a health measure and to 0.013 and 0.008 when PCS and MCS from the SF-36 instrument are used as health measures, respectively. This is in the vicinity of the estimate from van Doorslaer et al. (C = 0.009 for Denmark) where HUI was used as a health status measure.[1] Decomposing the concentration indices for EQ-5D and PCS gives surprisingly similar results. Inactivity in the labour market is important for income-related health inequality. Being retired is the biggest contributor to the inequality estimates. Income-inequality is also an important contributor to income-related inequality in health contrary to the findings in van Doorslaer et al. where almost all of the income-related inequality in health could be ascribed to being retired and where income practically played no role.[1] The age and gender variables contribute negatively to the inequality estimates. That is, the age and gender vector contributes in favour of the lower income groups and standardizing for these socio-demographic variables increases the inequality estimates. Education, marital status, and the health-related life-style factors play a minor role in explaining income-related health inequality – at least in this cross-sectional framework. With respect to different dimensions of health, having pain/discomfort or having reported health problems in general are important factors in explaining the size of income-related health inequality (using EQ-5D TTO-values).

Health care is in general concentrated among the lower income groups (C = -0.14 for aggregate health care). This pattern is present for all types of health care (significant concentration indices for hospital visits, prescription medicine, and GP consultations) except for dentistry where the services are concentrated among the higher income groups. Standardizing for age, gender, and health status to take need into account modifies the results somewhat. At the aggregate level the standardized concentration index is no longer significantly different from zero. In the primary health care sector the services are concentrated among the higher income groups when need is taken into account (significant standardized concentration indices for prescription medicine and dentistry). The unstandardized estimates are close to the estimates from van Doorslaer et al.[2] However, the standardized measures do deviate in some cases. The most important deviation is for specialist treatment where no income-related inequality is found in the present study. This is contrary to international results, including Denmark, where considerable income-related inequality in specialist treatment was found.[2,3] Inactivity in the labour market is also important for income-related inequality in health care. Being retired is the biggest contributor to the inequality estimates, but in favour of the lower income groups. Income is a positive contributor to income-related inequality in health care, that is, it increases the inequality estimate in favour of the higher income groups. However, the contribution is only significant for some types of health care, and not at the aggregate level. The need standardizing variables (age, gender, and health status) diminish the inequality estimates in most case. That is, the standardization increases the concentration indices in favour of the higher income groups. Education, marital status, and the health-related life-style factors play a minor role in explaining income-related inequality in health care – at least in this cross-sectional framework. The hospital sector constitutes 63 percent of the aggregate health care costs. Therefore, the hospital sector dominates the overall inequality measure. However, the contribution to overall income-related inequality in health care from the hospital sector is even bigger than what could be expected from the share of the aggregate health care costs (the inequality in hospital treatment contributes with 89 percent of overall concentration index).

Policy implications

The thesis has assessed the two principles: *equality in health* and *equal treatment for equal need*. Whether deviations from these principles are perceived as a problem that necessitates policy initiatives is a normative issue. The results can be used in a positive manner to obtain information about the distribution of health and health care and its relationship with socio-demographic and socio-economic variables, or the results can also be used in a normative manner to evaluate how well the principles have been met.

One problem of evaluating a principle is that society might have several objectives, which is clearly the case for the Danish health care sector as was pointed out in Chapter 1. If society aims at a trade-off between different objectives, say efficiency and equality in health, it is clearly problematic to evaluate the health care sector according to just one principle. Therefore, one has to be careful with interpretations of principle-fulfillment.

Assuming that a principle of an equal distribution is the first and foremost objective and the concentration index is found to be of considerable size, then the decomposition analysis can contribute with information about the importance of certain variables and relationships. The decomposition by determinants decomposes the concentration index into concentration indices for the different determinants weighted by elasticities.[4] The income-related inequality in either health or health care, represented by the concentration index, can therefore, in principle, be diminished by reducing the elasticity or the concentration index for a particular determinant.[1] The elasticity consists of the regression coefficient for the partial effect of the determinant on the variable of interest and the mean of the determinant, which is a proportion if the determinant is a represented by a dummy variable. Thus, the effect on income-related inequality in health or health care from a single characteristic depends on the proportion of people with that characteristic, its partial effect on the variable of interest (health or health care), and the distribution of the characteristic with respect to income groups.

The decomposition by dimension can contribute with information about the importance of the dimension to the overall income-related inequality. The importance of the dimension depends on the share of the variable of interest (health or health care) for this dimension of the aggregate level, and the income-related inequality in this dimension.

Even if obvious policy areas can be deduced from the results there can be many restrictions, such as ethical side-constraints, on implementing policies to combat violations of desired principles. Furthermore, the study contributes with information about the importance of determinants and dimensions for the distribution of health and health care. However, there is no information about the chance of successful intervention in these areas. Some areas might, for instance, be modifiable only by very cost-ineffective interventions[52].

With respect to income-related inequality in health, being retired is the biggest contributor, so it is natural to concentrate the attention on this characteristic. Its contribution is sizeable because the proportion of retired people is fairly large (19 percent), being retired is significantly correlated with lower health status (0.09 lower EQ-5D-score compared to the reference group of unskilled), and retired people are concentrated among the lower income groups ($C = -0.38$)[53]. The proportion of people being retired can be difficult to change as people are selected into retirement by old age and possibly also by bad health. Even if people could be moved into another category, such as a student or a worker, the health status would not automatically be improved, and the overall effect on the concentration index would remain the same. However, the income-related health inequality could be diminished by improving the health status of the retired or by redistributing income to improve the income position of the retired. The easiest technical solution to diminish the concentration index would probably be the redistribution of income. However, it is questionable whether this policy initiative is in the spirit of the principle of income-related equality in health. If the principle expresses the perception that health is a special good that requires special distributional concerns independently of income, then it might be perceived as goal displacement when income is modified to diminish income-related inequality in health[54]. The most relevant approach would simply be to improve the health status for the retired. The possibilities for improving the health status for this group of people are possibly limited by a high shadow price of health investments due to old age and low income. However, improving health for this group would probably not be completely impossible.

---

[52] Although equity and efficiency are seen as two separate objectives, it is hard to imagine that cost-effectiveness considerations would play no role in achieving equity objectives. There are opportunity costs even in the fulfillment of equity objectives.

[53] As the contribution depends on the dummy coefficient the size of the contribution is influenced by the choice of the reference category for the dummy vector.

[54] Although low income among the retired could, of course, be a concern in itself.

The other large contributor to income-related inequality in health is income itself. As pointed out in van Doorslaer et al. the income-related inequality in health is relatively high in Denmark despite the fact that the income inequality is fairly low relative to other European countries.[1] The contribution from income therefore stems from the significant positive correlation between income and health. Thus, the policy interventions should probably address this relationship rather than the income distribution per se.

The decomposition into dimensions shows that the pain/discomfort dimension is the biggest contributor. This is first and foremost due to the importance of pain and discomfort for the overall health status and not so much due to the distribution of pain/discomfort across income groups.

For income-related inequality in health care utilization the standardized concentration index is negative and insignificant. The specific types of health care are therefore of bigger interest for the policy initiatives. The concentration indices are large and positive for types of health care with high degrees of co-payment (Prescription medicine, dentistry, and physiotherapy). It is tempting to interpret the income-related inequality in these types of health care as being caused by a lower ability or willingness to pay for the lower income groups. For dentistry and physiotherapy, income does explain the vast majority of the positive contribution to the concentration indices. If the lower income groups face higher shadow prices for investments in health additional cost in the form of co-payment will probably only widen the gap even further. A natural policy implication is to reconsider the high co-payment rates for these services. For prescription medicine the income component only explains a small part of the positive contribution as most of it can be attributed to an unexplained component which makes it more difficult to interpret. For most of the dimensions being retired is a large contributor to the concentration indices. However, the contribution is negative, i.e. it diminishes the inequality in favour of the higher income groups. That is, the retired people, although concentrated among the lower income groups, do receive more health care services – perhaps to compensate them for their lower health status.

Limitations

As any other empirical study this thesis has some limitations and uncertainties. The following sections describe the most general problems encountered in the thesis. Some of the problems have already been dealt with in discussion sections in the previous chapters.

Focus of the study

The study focuses only on two types of inequality: *equality in health* and *equal treatment for equal need*. Only horizontal versions of these principles with regard to income position have been analyzed. As is clear from Chapter 1 distributional justice is a larger area than just these two principles. Other types of inequality could also have been studied. Most obvious is the use of other socio-economic variables as ranking variable. For instance, education or some index of socio-economic status could have been utilized to estimate other types of socio-economic inequality in health and health care. Furthermore, if inequality is perceived as a problem per se, independently of socio-economic status, then pure inequality measures, e.g. the Gini coefficient, could have been estimated by using health or health care as the ranking variable and variable of interest[55].[6] As the Gini-coefficient is a special case of the concentration index the decomposition techniques also apply to the Gini although attention has to be given to the ranking variable as it is not fixed across dimensions[56].

In the study, some aspects are ignored such as the relationship between the two principles of equality mentioned above. For example, what is the size of the income-related inequality in health

---

[55] The focus on pure inequality diminishes the violation of what Elster calls ethical individualism: The possibility that an individual in the name of equity will be discriminated due to group characteristics.[5] For example, if a rich person receives below average treatment because rich people in general receive too much health care compared to poor people. The variation is captured by the concentration index. However, given a positive concentration index for health care it is possible that some rich individuals receive less than average health care (given need).

[56] Contrary to the concentration index, where the ranking variable can be fixed, e.g. the income rank, across analyses of different variables the ranking variable for the Gini coefficient will vary with the variable analyzed.

care as measured in terms of improvements in health, or what is the size of the income-related inequality in health that can ascribed to utilization of health care? These questions are not at all straight-forward to analyze empirically. With respect to utilization of health care, the focus has only been on realized access. Potential access in the sense of opportunity to use has been disregarded[57]. In addition, there has been no investigation on the distributional aspects of health care finance[58].

Assumptions

Throughout the thesis it is assumed that health and health care are goods – as opposed to bads. That is, more is preferred to less. Although most people would agree with the notion that good-health is better than ill-health, it is less clear that more health care is always better than less health care. Health care is usually only consumed for the effect it has on health (or on utility). Health care per se is most often perceived as a bad rather than a good.[9-11] Furthermore, too much health care may in some situations have a negative effect on health.[12,13] However, this phenomenon should probably be classified as inappropriate health care rather than too much health care. More resources spent on health care for the individual, if correctly applied, would probably always have an expected non-negative effect on health status. In this study, however, it is impossible to distinguish between appropriate and inappropriate health care[59]. It is quite likely that some health care services do not

---

[57] Supply side variables could have been used in the analyses in various ways. For instance, proximity to health facilities or the number of doctors per capita in the area could have been used as a proxy for access costs (or for need) in the health care utilization functions.[7]

[58] If the first half of the Marxian dictum of "From each according to his ability – to each according to his needs" is applied to health care it means that health care should be financed according to ability to pay. However, as Wagstaff et al. have pointed out, as long as the financing of health care is separated from utilization at the point of delivery it is hard to justify this principle.[8] Perhaps health is a special good among other goods but is health care financing a special type of financing among the financing of all tax-financed goods?

[59] The data set is detailed enough for the possibilities of finding some of the inappropriate health care events For example, some adverse drug events could in principle be identified by applying certain rules to the utilization pattern. However, for the present study such analyses would be overwhelmingly comprehensive and

benefit the patients. The problem is particularly disturbing if some groups receive more inappropriate treatment than other groups. The issue makes it harder to interpret the inequality estimates. If the problem is of considerable size, then it is impossible to tell whether differentials in use of health care across groups imply that some groups get it right and others receive too little or if some groups get it right and others receive too much, or a combination of these two situations.

Another important assumption is the assumption that the average level of utilization given age, gender, and health status is the appropriate amount.[3,14,15] It is questionable whether the assumption is suitable if there is vertical inequity or if the problem of inappropriate health care is of considerable proportion. Likewise, if the health variable is not a valid proxy for need the average level of health care utilization will not in general be the correct one.

The cross-sectional design

The study design is a cross-sectional study design. The people participating have been interviewed only once when they were asked about health status, health behaviour, and socio-economic characteristics. Health care is not measured at one point in time but over the course of two years (2000 and 2001) as health care utilization is more easily measured as a flow concept than a stock concept. A period of two years has been chosen for several reasons. Two years is a period long enough to give a reliable estimate of health care utilization of the individual. The period is also long enough to diminish the zero-consumption problems and random fluctuations. Furthermore, the data collection for the interviews took place in the years 2000 and 2001, more specifically around the turn of the year into 2001. The health status indicators are point estimates, and will be less valid as standardization variables for health care consumption that has occurred too long before or after the time of the interview, it could have been an improvement to narrow the period down to a smaller time interval around the data collection. However, the missing date variable for a large number of the health care services (data from the National Health

---

it would only reveal a part of the problem. Furthermore, inappropriate health care due to wrong diagnoses and the like would be impossible to identify.

Insurance Service Registry) made it necessary to work with years as discrete units.

The period of two years of the collection of health care data is long enough for attrition due to death to take place. Individuals who died in the period from the time where the sample was drawn to the time of interview have naturally been excluded from the sample. It is possible that some of the respondents have died since the time of interview (or left Funen County for other reasons). As there is no information about this characteristic these respondents are included in the working sample. Had the information been available it is not clear whether these respondents should have been included or excluded in the analyses. In any case it is a question concerning very few respondents.

Working with cross-sectional data naturally invokes the question about causal interpretations. As there is no time sequence of events we cannot be sure of the direction of causality. It is possible that there is some simultaneity in the relationship between health and health care and that the values of some explanatory variables are determined by health status rather than the other way around, or health and the explanatory variables are correlated with unobserved characteristics.[1,16] Therefore, causal interpretations should be done with caution. Gross income is from the previous year (1999) so it can obviously not be determined by instantaneous health status or health care utilization in 2000 and 2001. However, the variables can possibly be jointly determined by unobserved characteristics. For estimation of health care utilization the data could have been limited to the year 2001 to improve the time sequence of health and health care. However, some of the respondents do have their health measured in 2001, so the attempt to create a time sequence to diminish the risk of simultaneity would not be perfect.

The health care variable

Health care utilization was measured as the costs of health care services and approximated by prices, charges or fees in monetary terms. Health care needs operationalization of some sort and using a common unit of measurement such as costs has some advantages. The different health services could be added together to an aggregate measure of health care utilization – between and within the different dimensions of health care.

In addition, the cost of a service represents the quality or importance of the procedure, although quality with regard to how the specific service has been carried out by the individual physician or surgeon is not captured by the size of the cost. Furthermore, using costs reminds us that there are opportunity costs of achieving equity principles. It is, however, important to bear in mind that prices, charges, and fees are only crude approximations of the costs and do not necessarily represent the shadow prices of the services.[17,18]

The aggregate measure of health care utilization has been classified into six types of health care: Use of somatic hospitals, GP, physiotherapy, dentistry, and prescription medicine. Other ways of categorizing health care was also possible. Hospital services could have been categorized into inpatient stays ambulatory visits, and emergency room visits. Additionally, a distinction between acute and elective treatment was possible. For the primary health care data additional categorization is less obvious although specific information on the different services was available to make it possible to analyze the distribution of certain special services. The level of aggregation was chosen to minimize the problems of substitutionability between the services, which makes it harder to interpret results (if, for instance, positive inequality in one type of service is off-set by negative inequality in another). The same treatments can be carried out, for example, as inpatient stays or ambulatory visits. However, as long as this is kept in mind a further disaggregation than the chosen one could have been useful. Besides, the chosen categorization into six types of health care is not completely exempt from the problem of substitutionability.

The health variable

Health status was used in the analyses for two reasons: As a proxy for need in the standardization procedure for the inequality estimates of health care utilization and as a measure of health for the health inequality estimates.

As a proxy for need the EQ-5D TTO value was used in most cases. The use of the EQ-5D value as a proxy for need is problematic in several ways. First of all, it is an instantaneous measure of health that is used as a proxy for need for health care for a longer period of time. The appropriateness of using this measure then depends on whether it can be interpreted as a measure of health status in general that is more or less constant over time, say a higher depreciation rate, or whether it refers to specific illnesses that vary from time to time with respect to severity and can possibly be cured by health care. The risk of simultaneity is bigger if the latter situation is the case. In addition, some health care services are utilized for the expected preventive effect. When treatment cures the illnesses the need for health care is not accounted for by the health status measure, which might show good or perfect health as a result of the treatment.

Another problem is the fact that one health status measure is used as a proxy for need for six types of health care. One measure obviously works better as a need-proxy for some types of health care than others. For dental care, for instance, the EQ-5D values seem to be particularly inappropriate as general health status cannot be expected to be a good proxy for dental health status. The EQ-5D TTO value summarizes the descriptive EQ-5D system into a single index given preferences of the general population for the trade-off between length of life and quality of life. Alternatively, the descriptive system could have been applied directly in the standardization specification with dummy variables for each dimension for having some or severe problems (or variables for each dimension with the TTO-coefficients as values). That way each dimension would play a role in the standardization procedure rather than only through the aggregate health measure. However, it is not clear that the specific dimensions would improve the prediction of need for services such as dental care.

Previously it has been shown that the inclusion of more than one health variable can decrease the inequality estimates as more health variables provide more information on aspects that determine health care utilization.[15,19] In the present study two indices of health status were available: EQ-5D and SF-36 (the question of general self-assessed health is included in the SF-36 descriptive system). The two descriptive systems explain more or less the same aspects of health. Therefore only one health index was used at a time.

Using health status as a measure of health for the health inequality estimates also presents some difficulties. As health status was only measured at one point in time it is a point estimate of the individuals' health status over a life course. The question is whether we are interested in just a point estimate of individual health or whether we are interested in health over a period of time, for example the quality adjusted length of life.[20] Using EQ-5D TTO values for good-health (as opposed to ill-health) the inequality is relative small compared to the average level, as most people are relatively close to 1. However, over a life course these small differences can accumulate to considerable differences, especially if the inequality constitutes length of life as well as quality of life.[21] Furthermore, the health measures rest on the assumption that people have the same understanding of health across socio-economic groups.[3,22-25] It is possible that, for instance, the lower income groups have a more pessimistic view of their life in general and therefore also of their health status. The opposite can also be the case if the higher income groups underestimate their good health or the lower income groups underestimate their bad health due to adaptation. However, unless we have a more objective measure of need we cannot quantify this reference bias.

The Danish TTO model does make it possible to obtain negative values for the EQ-5D score and they represent health states that are valued worse than death.[26] The EQ-5D score is, as a matter of fact, not a ratio-scaled variable as there is no natural lower limit for how undesirable a health state can be in comparison to death.[18] In principle, the concentration index is appropriate only for ratio-scaled variables.[27] However, as only five respondents had negative values and death seems to be a natural zero point, the problem of negative values has been ignored.

There are no negative values in the PCS and MCS variables. However, using the concentration index on these variables is no less disturbing. Negative values were avoided by adding 50 to the PCS and MCS scales. As the concentration index is affected by adding a constant, the addition of 50 appears somewhat arbitrary, and it is questionable whether the PCS and MCS scales are ratio-scaled variables. However, it was outside the scope of the study to assess the scoring mechanism for the SF-36 summary scores and the PCS and MCS scores have been taken as given.

The income variable

Income was chosen as the socio-economic ranking variable. The income variable was taken from the health survey. The respondents were posed questions about their personal gross income in 1999 (gross of tax and deductibles). The validity of using this variable depends on what we want to measure. Are we interested in income as a measure of socio-economic status or a measure of the material conditions that may influence health and ability to pay? The self-reported gross income variable is to some extent an imperfect measure for both of these perspectives.

Income is not wealth. Income can fluctuate over time and low income in 1999 might reflect neither low socio-economic status nor ability to pay. Gross income in Denmark does reflect transfers for the receiver but not for the contributor. Disposable income, income net of tax and deductible, would be a better approximation of ability to pay. In some studies household income is used, as ability to pay or socio-economic position is not necessarily an individual phenomenon.[1-3,14,15,28] Household income information was not available for the present study, although information about family structure and marital status did exist among the variables in the database.

Income is a sensitive question in health surveys and a large fraction of the respondents was reluctant to answer that question in the Funen County Health Survey. Four hundred eighty five respondents were left out of the analysis due to missing observations with regard to income. Item non-response was not examined in the non-response analysis in Chapter 7. However, additional non-response analyses have shown that item non-response due to income is a considerable and important contributor to the non-response bias in health care utilization in a downward direction. In addition, the income answers could be subject to recall bias as not all respondents might remember (or be honest about) their exact gross income from the previous year. On the other hand, income was given in income categories and the concentration indices might not be that sensitive to the precision of the income. Descriptive statistics of the income variable were compared to income statistics from register based data and there were no signs of considerable deviations.

Econometric specifications

To predict utilization of health care a two-part model was used to address the problem of zero-consumption observations for a considerable part of the population and the skewness of the distribution. By applying the two-part model the question of use or not use is separated from the level of utilization for the individuals who are users.[29-31] The two parts have been estimated separately and this approach rests on the assumption that the decision to use and the decision about the level of utilization are actually independent. However, even if the two decisions are actually two detached choices they can both be correlated with the same unobservable variables.[30] This phenomenon, if present, suggests that a specification with a joint determination of use or no use and the level of utilization could be more appropriate. The review by Jones shows that there is some disagreement with respect to the choice between two-part models and selection models.[30]

In the second part of the two-part model the logarithm was taken of the dependent variable – the health care variable – to diminish the skewness of the data.[31,32] To retransform predicted values into the original scale the non-parametric smearing estimator was applied. The smearing estimator is redundant when the predictions are used for the indirect standardization approach. Only the relative level of utilization (utilization relative to the mean) is needed for the concentration index, as the concentration index is insensitive to relative changes and the smearing estimator is a constant scaling up all predicted observations. However, when using the decomposition approach by approximating linear marginal effects by average partial effects the smearing estimator has been used to retransform the predicted values into the original scales.[33] The non-parametric smearing estimator is a consistent estimator, however, only insofar as the regression coefficients do not depend on the explanatory variables.[29,30,32,34] Regression diagnostics indicate that there is still potential heteroskedasticity in several of the utilization models even after removing some of the skewness by the log transformation. This could potentially bias the smearing estimators and therefore also influence the average partial effects. Interpretations of the average partial effects as approximations of linear marginal effects should therefore be done with caution.

The EQ-5D variables also present skewed distributions as 60 percent of the population have perfect health. That is, the distribution is left-skewed. The two-part model is not an obvious choice for a model for health status prediction, partly because health is concentrated at the upper end of the scale and partly because there are not two separate mechanisms to explain as in the utilization model. The concentration at 1 (perfect health) should rather be perceived as a censoring in this point. A selection model such as the tobit model would therefore be more appropriate to address the problem of concentration of people with perfect health. However, the subdimensions of EQ-5D (weighted by TTO weights) each has only three levels. Given this fact it was therefore judged that the tobit model would not necessarily be an improvement of the specification compared to an OLS model. After all, the decomposition technique is based on OLS regression.[4] OLS regression models were therefore applied to the decomposition of the EQ-5D concentration index. For future work a selection model could be considered for predicting EQ-5D values.

The values from the SF-36 summary scores do not show the same problems with floor or ceiling effects, although some of the subscales do have the values concentrated at the higher end. For convenience, OLS regressions were applied to health status predictions to be used in the decomposition techniques.

Generalizability

The analyses in the study have been based on a stratified survey sample of 5,000 individuals who were randomly selected within the strata. If sample weights are used the study should be representative for the Funen County population at the time of data collection[60]. A number of problems may have influenced the representativity.

The parent population where the sample has been extracted from is not complete. People can choose to be registered as exempt from research projects in the Centralised Civil Register. According to Linde, about 10 percent of the population is registered with this exemption and this could possible threaten the otherwise random selection of

---

[60] Although statistical uncertainty is always present when a sample is drawn randomly from a parent population.

individuals for the sample population.[35] The extent of the problem around the time of data collection is not well known, although we do know that the problem has increased over time, so it was most likely smaller than 10 percent in 2000.

Another threat to the representativity is the problem of non-response. A non-response analysis of the non-response bias for the health care utilization estimates is presented in Chapter 7. Due to the purpose of the chapter of comparing two health surveys the focus is strictly on unit non-response. However, due to the large number of respondents who failed to answer certain questions in the survey, in particularly the income question, the item non-response turned out to be considerable (ten percent of the sampled population). This would not necessarily be a big problem for the representativity if item non-respondents did not deviate from the rest of the respondents.[36,37] However, the effect of item non-response on the health care utilization estimates is substantial. Unit non-response decreases the aggregate health care estimate by about DKK 1,000 and item non-response further decreases it by about DKK 1,000, so that the estimate for the interviewed is close to DKK 18,000, or about 10 percent lower than the "true" estimate (of all the sampled individuals). We know that the non-respondents utilize more health care and the item non-respondents have a lower level of (self-reported) education than the respondents, so they probably also have a lower health status and make less money. However, it is not easy to guess the size and direction of the bias on the inequality estimates as these measures are bivariate estimates.

Bearing in mind that there are potential problems with non-response and a completely randomized selection procedure the findings of the study can be generalized to the Funen County population at the time of data collection. The question is whether the results can be generalized to a wider geographical area or to a different point in time. At the time of the data collection the Danish health care system was a relatively decentralized system with the county governments having political, economic, and operational responsibility of the local health care systems.[38-40] This could potentially lead to local differences in the service level.[40] However, free choice of hospitals in Denmark for certain procedures regardless of county of residence for the patient, political pressure, guidelines and legislation at the national level have possibly reduced the potential heterogeneity. Furthermore, the general structure of co-payment for different types of health care services was the same across counties. As Funen County was fairly similar to the rest of Denmark with respect to some key figures regarding demographic characteristics and health care utilization a generalization to the rest of Denmark would probably be quite justifiable. This is supported by previous studies, based on Denmark, with overall results that are reasonably similar.[1-3]

With respect to the time dimension, some years have passed since the data collection took place. The Danish health care system is known for its longitudinal stability. For a long period of time only gradual adjustments have taken place and the system has been devoid of actual health care reforms. As of January 2007, a reform has been launched.[39,40] The reform has changed the political decentralization structure but the principles of access and co-payment have remained the same. Funen County no longer exists as a political unit although the geographical area is, of course, still there. The major findings in the study are most likely still prevailing in the Danish or Funen health care system in 2007. The long run consequences of the reform are more difficult to predict. Another important aspect in the Danish health care system is the increasing use of supplementary for-profit health care insurance, most often provided by employers as a fringe benefit to the employees.[40] At the time of data collection the prevalence of these insurance schemes was very limited. However, they are now becoming increasingly common among those who are active in the labour market. If the increasing use of private insurance is a slippery slope towards more private financing of health care services this could have an important impact on the future arrangements for the Danish health care system. Future research must show the effect on access to health care and on the distribution of health and health care.

Future research

Future research points in three directions. First of all, the study was carried out within a limited geographical area of Denmark. This was due to the fact that for the present study survey data was only available for Funen County. Comprehensive national health surveys do exist and have also been merged with registers (for example the Danish Health

Interview survey 2000).[41,42] When updating the present analyses an obvious choice would be to use a national survey and to merge it with registers including health care utilization and socio-demographic and socio-economic variables. Access to such data could improve the studies in several ways. 1) The data quality would be improved by having more socio-economic variables such as income (or household income) and education from registers. This would improve the accuracy of the variables and diminish the risk of recall bias, reporting bias and item non-response bias[61]. 2) More types of health care can be extracted from national registers such as contacts at psychiatric hospitals and prescription medicine not entitled to reimbursement and this would make the aggregate measure of health care utilization more complete.[44,45] 3) Surveys such as the Danish Health Interview Survey contain questions about health care utilization and these could be used to supplement the register based estimates with information on health care utilization that cannot be extracted from registers such as use of over-the-counter medicine and treatment by therapists outside the general health service system (reflexology, acupuncture, natural medicinal products etc.) although information on this kind of utilization will exhibit the normal problems of self-reported use of health care services.[41] 4) A comprehensive health survey with a richer set of health variables would increase the availability of appropriate need proxies for specific types of health care utilization (e.g. dental health care). 5) If several periods are available from a survey and the registers the used of lagged variables and panel data techniques can be used to address some of the problems with endogeneity.[46]

Another area for future research is pure inequality in health. Measures of pure inequality capture the inequality no matter how it is distributed with respect to socio-economic position. As people naturally differ with regard to socio-demographic characteristics and other

---

[61] More variables from registers could also improve non-response analysis as more information would be available for respondents and non-respondents. With inspiration from Oaxaca the bias components in Chapter 7 could, for instance, be further decomposed into components from differences in characteristics and components due to differences in behaviour.[43] Preliminary analyses have been carried out on data from the Funen County Health Survey but there are problems with lack of relevant variables as well as appropriate specifications.

features that are perceived as acceptable correlates with health the pure inequality measures might not be so interesting per se. However, an explanation of the sources of pure inequality in health could have some policy relevance. The pure inequality measure, the health Gini-coefficient, could be decomposed into a component of socio-economic inequality in health and a component of rank differences between health and the socio-economic variable as shown by Wagstaff et al.[6] Alternatively, the health Gini-coefficient could be decomposed into a sum of concentration indices for explanatory variables weighted by health elasticities with respect to the explanatory variables.[4] This decomposition is equivalent to the one applied in Chapter 5 but with health status used as a ranking variable in lieu of income. Pure inequality would then be explained by sources from various explanatory variables. However, there would be no component of pure income-inequality. Income would be represented by a concentration index of income with respect to the ranking of health. Another problem is the ranking variable that will differ across dimensions unless the overall ranking variable is fixed across dimensions, such that the subdimensions are represented by concentration indices of inequality in subdimensional health with respect to the ranking variable of overall health. Whether these changes are appropriate or perhaps an improvement compared to the analyses of socio-economic inequality in health depends on the focus and purpose of the study.

A third area for attention is the question about the relevant health variable for measuring income-related inequality in health. In Chapter 5 the EQ-5D value was used as a health status measure. However, this value is in principle only a point estimate of health. Health measured over a period of time might be seen as a more adequate variable. For example, the focus could be on lifetime health such as the number of QALYs over a lifetime.[20] Using this focus for estimating income-related inequality is not straight-forward as it is associated with some difficulties and choices. To measure lifetime health for a cohort would take a lifetime. Although interestingly enough per se, the policy relevance would be limited by the fact that it would not characterize the present population (but rather past populations or future populations if the study design is prospective). Another approach would be to use expected future quality adjusted length of life. In some studies Cox proportional hazard models have been used on censored survival time of cohorts to estimate life expectancy adjusted for health-related quality for different groups.[21,47] Another strategy would be to use life table techniques to estimate quality adjusted life-expectancy for different socio-economic groups. An advantage of using life table techniques is that only data for a short period of time is required. However, the approach is also connected with some difficulties. What variables should be used to distinguish between different groups? Is it possible and does it make sense to estimate lifetime expected income to be used as a ranking variable? Should past health somehow be added to the estimates of quality adjusted life-expectancy along the lines of the *fair innings* argument?[20] Furthermore, given the simulation-oriented approach to measuring lifetime health it would be much more difficult to maintain individual variability let alone carry out decompositions of the sources of lifetime-income-related inequality in quality adjusted length of life. Future research must show how far we can go in this area. The rich availability of surveys and registers in Denmark and the possibilities of combining them is probably not the worst starting-point for research in this area.

Conclusion

In this thesis concentration indices were used to estimate income-related inequality in the distribution of health and health care in Funen County, Denmark in 2000 and 2001. Decomposition techniques were applied to the concentration indices to obtain information on the composition and sources of inequality from determinants and dimensions. The analyses were carried out using a database consisting of a health survey and various registers. The health survey consisted of information on health status, health behaviour, and socio-economic characteristics. The registers consisted of information on health care utilization such as visits at the hospital and services in the primary health care sector i.e. visits at the general practitioner (GP), specialist practitioner, dentist, physiotherapist, and utilization of prescription medicine. The database consisted of 5,000 individuals with permanent address in Funen County. However, due to oversampling, external and internal non-response only 2,915 individuals were available for the analyses.

A review of the health equity literature showed that the views on distributional justice are numerous and multifarious among researchers, policy-makers, and the general population. This thesis has evaluated only two aspects of distributional justice: *Equal treatment for equal need* and *equality in health*. Both principles have been evaluated with respect to income to assess whether individuals with different income position are equally well-off with regard to utilization of health care and current health status.

Health care is often seen as a special good because of its instrumentality in producing good health. The analyses showed that health care, measured as health care costs, is in general concentrated among the lower income groups. The concentration index for aggregate health care has been estimated to -0.14. This pattern is present for almost all types of health care and is significant for concentration indices of hospital visits, prescription medicine, and GP consultations. One exception is dentistry where the services are concentrated among the higher income groups.

The concentration indices have been standardized for age, gender, and health status. These variables have been used as a proxy for need for health care in the evaluation of *equal treatment for equal need*. The standardization modifies the results somewhat. At the aggregate level the need-standardization of the concentration index makes the inequality estimate statistically insignificant. That is, the principle of *equal treatment of equal need* does not seem to be violated for overall health care utilization.

The hospital sector constitutes the majority of the aggregate health care costs. Therefore, the concentration index for the hospital sector dominates the overall inequality measure. However, the contribution to overall income-related inequality in health care from the hospital sector is even bigger than what could be expected from the share of the aggregate health care costs.

In the primary health care sector need-standardized concentration indices indicate that the services are concentrated among the higher income groups. This is especially true for services with a high degree of co-payment. The standardized concentration indices for prescription medicine and dentistry are statistically significant. Contrary to international findings, the income-related inequality in specialist treatment is small and insignificant.

Among the determinants, income inequality contributes to income-related inequality in health care utilization in favour of the higher income groups. However, the contribution is only significant for some types of health care, and not at the aggregate level. For prescription medicine most of the positive inequality is attributed to an unexplained component and the direct effect of income plays only a minor role. Inactivity in the labour market is also an important variable. Being retired is the biggest contributor to the inequality estimates, but in a downward direction, that is, in favour of the lower income groups. Education, marital status, and the health-related life-style factors play a minor role in explaining income-related inequality in health care.

Equality in health is sometimes seen as the ultimate aim of distributional justice as good health is a necessity for individuals to flourish as human beings and to enjoy all the good things in life. The results showed that good health is concentrated among the higher income groups. The concentration index has been estimated to 0.013 for health status represented by EQ-5D values.

Among determinants, inactivity in the labour market is important for income-related health inequality. Being retired is the biggest contributor to the inequality estimates. Income-inequality is also an important contributor to income-related inequality in health contrary to previous results for Denmark. The age and gender variables contribute negatively to the inequality estimates. That is, if the concentration indices are standardized for socio-demographic variables then the inequality estimate will increase. Education, marital status, and the health-related life-style factors play a minor role in explaining income-related health inequality. With respect to different dimensions of health, having pain/discomfort or having reported health problems in general are important health dimensions in explaining the size of income-related health inequality.

The analyses were also carried out with the SF-36 component scores for physical and mental health (PCS and MCS). The concentration indices were estimated to 0.013 and 0.008 for PCS and MCS, respectively. Decomposing the concentration indices for EQ-5D and PCS gives surprisingly similar results. The decomposition of the concentration index for MCS is somewhat different as age and gender contribute positively – in favour of the higher income groups – and activity in the labour market plays a smaller role. The complicated scoring mechanism of the SF-36 components scores makes the decomposition into health dimensions difficult to interpret.

The thesis shows that decompositions can be useful when using concentration indices to estimate income-related inequality in health and health care. Different determinants and dimensions contribute to the overall inequality estimate with varying degrees and the decomposition methodology can assist with pointing out the importance and off-setting effects of different factors. However, the possibility and the appropriateness of modifying the different factors cannot be deduced from this kind of analysis. Furthermore, the analyses from the present thesis were carried out as a cross-sectional design. Therefore, causal interpretations have to be done with caution.

References

1. van Doorslaer E, Koolman X. Explaining the differences in income-related health inequalities across European countries. *Health Econ* 2004;**13**:609-28.

2. van Doorslaer E, Masseria C, and the OECD Health Equity Research Group Members. Income-Related Inequality in the Use of Medical Care in 21 OECD Countries. 14. 2004. Paris, OECD. OECD Health working papers.

3. van Doorslaer E, Koolman X, Jones AM. Explaining income-related inequalities in doctor utilisation in Europe. *Health Econ* 2004;**13**:629-47.

4. Wagstaff A, van Doorslaer E, Watanabe N. On Decomposing the Causes of Health Sector Inequalities with an Application to Malnutrition Inequalities in Vietnam. *J Econometrics* 2003;**112**:207-23.

5. Elster J. *Local Justice: How Institutions Allocate Scarce Goods and Necessary* Burdens.Russell Sage Foundation, 1992.

6. Wagstaff A, van Doorslaer E. Overall versus socioeconomic health inequality: a measurement framework and two empirical illustrations. *Health Econ* 2004;**13**:297-301.

7. Morris S, Sutton M, Gravelle H. Inequity and inequality in the use of health care in England: an empirical investigation. *Soc Sci Med* 2005;**60**:1251-66.

8. Wagstaff A, van Doorslaer E. Equity in Health Care Finance and Delivery. *Handbook of health economics.Volume 1B* 2000;1803-62.

9. Grossman M. The Human Capital Model. *Handbook of health economics. Volume 1A* 2000;347-408.

10. Hurley J. An Overview of the Normative Economics of the Health Sector. *Handbook of health economics. Volume 1A* 2000;55-118.

11. Hurley J. Ethics, economics, and public financing of health care. *J Med Ethics* 2001;**27**:234-39.

12. Culyer AJ, Wagstaff A. Equity and Equality in Health and Health Care. *J Health Econ* 1993;**12**:431-57.

13. Beijer HJ, de Blaey CJ. Hospitalisations caused by adverse drug reactions (ADR): a meta-analysis of observational studies. *Pharm World Sci* 2002;**24**:46-54.

14. Bleichrodt H, van Doorslaer E. A welfare economics foundation for health inequality measurement. *J Health Econ* 2006;**25**:945-57.

15. van Doorslaer E, Wagstaff A, van der Burg H, Christiansen T, De Graeve D, Duchesne I, Gerdtham UG, Gerfin M, Geurts J, Gross L, Häkkinen U, John J, Klavus J, Leu RE, Nolan B, O'Donnell O, Propper C, Puffer F, Schellhorn M, Sundberg G, Winkelhake O. Equity in the delivery of health care in Europe and the US. *J Health Econ* 2000;**19**:553-83.

16. Smith JP. Healthy bodies and thick wallets: the dual relation between health and economic status. *Journal of Economic Perspectives* 1999;**13**:145-66.

17. Brouwer W, Rutten F, Koopmanschap M. Costing in economic evaluation. In: Drummond M.F., McGuire A, editors. *Economic Evaluation in Health Care*. Oxford University Press, 2001.

18. Drummond MF, O'Brien B, Stoddart GL, Torrance GW. *Methods for the Economic Evaluation of Health Care Programmes.* Second Edition ed.Oxford University Press, 1997.

19. Christiansen T. *Equity in the Delivery of Health Care in Denmark.* CHS Working Paper. University of Southern Denmark 1997;**10**.

20. Williams A. Intergenerational equity: an exploration of the 'fair innings' argument. *Health Econ* 1997;**6**:117-32.

21. Burström K, Johannesson M, Diderichsen F. Increasing socio-economic inequalities in life expectancy and QALYs in Sweden 1980-1997. *Health Econ* 2005;**14**:831-50.

22. Groot W. Adaptation and scale of reference bias in self-assessments of quality of life
J Health Econ 2000;**19**:403-20.

23. Jürges H. *Self-assessed health, reference points, and mortality.* MEA Discussion Paper 57-04. 2005.

24. van Doorslaer E, Gerdtham UG. Does inequality in self-assessed health predict inequality in survival by income? Evidence from Swedish data. *Soc Sci Med* 2003;**57**:1621-29.

25. Kaplan G, Baron-Epel O. What lies behind the subjective evaluation of health status? *Soc Sci Med* 2003;**56**:1669-76.

26. Wittrup-Jensen KU, Lauridsen JT, Gudex C, Brooks R, and Pedersen KM. Estimating danish EQ-5D tariffs using the time trade-off (TTO) and visual analogue scale (VAS) methods. In Norinder AL, Pedersen KM, Roos P (eds) *Proceedings of the 18th Plenary Meeting of the EuroQol Group, 6th - 7th September, 2001*, Copenhagen, Denmark, IHE- The Swedish Institute for Health Economics, Lund. 2001.

27. Clarke PM, Gerdtham UG, Johannesson M, Bingefors K, Smith L. On the measurement of relative and absolute income-related health inequality. *Soc Sci Med.* 2002;**55**:1923-28.

28. van Doorslaer E, Wagstaff A, Bleichrodt H et al. Income-related inequalities in health: some international comparisons. *J Health Econ* 1997;**16**:93-112.

29. Manning WG, Newhouse JP, Duan N, Keeler EB, Leibowitz A. Health Insurance and the Demand for Medical Care: Evidence from a randomized Experiment. *American Econ Rev* 1987;**77**:251-77.

30. Jones AM. Health Econometrics. *Handbook of health economics. Volume 1A.* 2000;265-345.

31. Lipscomb J, Ancukiewicz M, Parmigiani G, Hasselblad V, Samsa G, Matchar DB. Predicting the cost of illness: a comparison of alternative models applied to stroke. *Med Decis Making* 1998;**18**:S39-S56.

32. Manning WG. The logged dependent variable, heteroscedasticity, and the retransformation problem. *J Health Econ* 1998;**17**:283-95.

33. Duan N. Smearing Estimate: A Nonparametric Retransformation Method. *J American Stat Assoc* 1983;**78**:605-10.

34. Mullahy J. Much ado about two: reconsidering retransformation and the two-part model in health econometrics. *J Health Econ* 1998;**17**:247-81.

35. Linde P. Web-undersøgelser og nye udfordringer til surveys. In: *Symposium i anvendt statistik.* Odense: Statistics Denmark & Department of Economics, University of Southern Denmark, 2005:77-88.

36. Greene WH. *Econometric Analysis*. 4 ed. Prentice Hall, 2000.

37. Groves RM, Couper MP. *Nonresponse in Household Interview Surveys*. Wiley Interscience, 1998.

38. Vallgårda S, Krasnik A, Vrangbæk K. Health Care Systems in Transition: Denmark. Thomson S, Mossialos E. 2001. *European Observatory on Health Care Systems. Health Care Systems in Transition*.

39. Vrangbæk K, Christiansen T. Health Policy in Denmark: Leaving the Decentralized Welfare Path? *J Health Politics, Policy and Law* 2005;**30**:29-52.

40. Pedersen KM, Christiansen T, Bech M. The Danish health care system: evolution - not revolution - in a decentralized system. *Health Econ* 2005;**14**:S41-S57.

41. Kjøller M, Rasmussen NK. Sundhed og sygelighed I Danmark 2000 .... & udviklingen siden 1987 [Danish Health and Morbidity Survey 2000 .... & trends since 1989]. 2002. National Institute of Public Health.

42. Helweg-Larsen K, Kjoller M, Davidsen M, Rasmussen NK, Madsen M. The Danish National Cohort Study (DANCOS). *Dan Med Bull* 2003;**50**:177-80.

43. Oaxaca RL. Male-female wage differentials in urban labor markets. *Int Econ Rev* 1973;**14**:693-709.

44. Munk-Jorgensen P, Mortensen M. Det Psykiatriske Centrale Forskningsregisters rolle i udforskningen af psykiatriske folkesygdomme [The role of Danish Psychiatric Central Research Registry in the research of widespread mental disorders]. *Ugeskr Laeger* 2004;**166**:1454-58.

45. Hallas J. Conducting pharmacoepidemiologic research in Denmark. *Pharmacoepidemiol Drug Saf* 2001;**10**:619-23.

46. Van Ourti T. Measuring horizontal inequity in Belgian health care using a Gaussian random effects two part count data model. *Health Econ* 2004;**13**:705-24.

47. Gerdtham UG, Johannesson M. Income-related inequality in life-years and quality-adjusted life-years. *J Health Econ* 2000;**19**:1007-26.

Dansk sammenfatning
(Danish summary)

Dansk sammenfatning

Baggrund
Fordelingsmæssige hensyn spiller en stor rolle for sundhedsvæsenets indretning og organisering. Den pågældende afhandling handler om, hvordan sundhed og sundhedsydelser rent faktisk er fordelt i befolkningen, og hvilke faktorer der kan påvirke disse fordelinger. Der er mange forskellige og ofte modstridende målsætninger med sundhedsvæsenet. Først og fremmest vil målsætningen ofte være at forbedre sundheden mest muligt og at forebygge og behandle sygdom. Dette oversættes af sundhedsøkonomer til en efficiensmålsætning om at maksimere sundheden eller nytten af sundhed i befolkningen. Der vil typisk også være nogle lighedsmålsætninger om en retfærdig fordeling af sundheden eller sundhedsydelserne. Dette begrundes hyppigt med, at sundhedsydelser bør ses som specielle goder, der kræver særlige fordelingsmæssige hensyn, idet sundhedsydelser er vigtige i produktionen af et godt helbred. Et godt helbred er videre en forudsætning for, at man som individ kan blomstre og tage aktiv del i alle livets goder.

Hvis sundhedsydelser ses som et specielt gode, der kræver særlige fordelingsmæssige hensyn, så er motivationen bag de fordelingsmæssige tiltag et vigtigt aspekt. Hvis motivationen er altruisme, så kan tiltagene begrundes af præferencer for et godt helbred for vores medmennesker. Da motivationen afhænger af præferencer, betragter økonomer denne tilgang som et spørgsmål om efficiens og kan i princippet indbygges i økonomiske modeller for maksimering af nytten af sundhed i befolkningen. En anden motivation er social retfærdighed, der bygger på tilslutning til principper, der vurderet fra en upartisk vinkel bedømmes som værende retfærdige.

Lighedsmålsætninger motiveret i social retfærdighed kan komme til udtryk på mange forskellige måder. Et fælles træk er dog, at "noget" skal være lige. Hvad dette "noget" er, vil typisk variere fra tilgang til tilgang. Utilitaristerne vil understrege, at nytten af sundhed og sundhedsydelser tæller lige meget, uanset hvem den tilfalder i maksimeringen af nytten i befolkningen. Dette ses dog ofte mere som en efficiensmålsætning end en lighedsmålsætning. En anden tilgang er, at forskellige individers sundhed ikke nødvendigvis tæller lige meget. F.eks. kan selvforskyldt dårligt helbred betyde, at man har gjort sig mindre fortjent til sundhedsydelser, eller at man har gjort sig fortjent til højere selvfinansiering. Libertarianerne fokuserer først og fremmest på lige individuelle rettigheder og friheder. Sundhedsydelser betragtes på lige fod med andre goder i samfundet, og en retfærdig fordeling eksisterer, hvis individuelle rettigheder ikke er blevet krænket. Rawlsianere ønsker en samfundsindretning, hvor institutioner skal sikre, at basale frihedsrettigheder er ligeligt fordelt, og hvor samfundet ellers er indrettet, så det gavner de dårligst stillede mest muligt. Oprindeligt var rawlsianske teorier ikke tiltænkt sundhedsspørgsmål, men er af nogle indarbejdet, så institutionerne skal sikre et normalt funktionsniveau for individerne, så de kan være funktionsdygtige medlemmer af samfundet. Egalitære teorier anvendt på sundhedsområdet fokuserer på lighed i sundhed eller sundhedsydelser. Forskellige principper har været appliceret: Det har været foreslået, at der skal gives *lige behandling for lige behov*. Implikationen af dette princip afhænger af definitionen af behov, som kan tage flere former, og vil ikke nødvendigvis føre til lighed i sundhed. Hvis autonomi vægtes højt, så omskrives princippet ofte til *lige adgang for lige behov*, således at det er *muligheden* for konsumere sundhedsydelser, der er det centrale. Da sundhedsydelser typisk forbruges for deres instrumentalitet i produktionen af sundhed, ses *lige sundhed* i befolkningen af nogle som den ultimative lighedsmålsætning.

Lighedsprincipper kan i de fleste tilfælde defineres i to versioner: *horisontal lighed* og *vertikal lighed*. Horisontal lighed betyder, at lige personer behandles lige, mens vertikal lighed vil sige, at forskellige personer skal behandles tilpas forskelligt. Den sidstnævnte type lighed kan være svær at håndtere, da det kræver en præcisering af, hvad der menes med tilpas forskelligt. Horisontal ulighed kan undersøges i forhold til karakteristika, som ikke bør have indflydelse på lige behandling. Hvis sundhedsområdet ses som et specielt område, der kræver specielle fordelingsmæssige hensyn uafhængigt af den generelle fordeling af goder i samfundet, så bør indkomst ikke spille en rolle (eller kun spille en begrænset rolle) i allokeringen sundhed og sundhedsydelser. I afhandlingen er der undersøgt to egalitære principper for fordeling af sundhed og sundhedsydelser i forhold til indkomst: *lige behandling for lige behov* og *lige sundhed*.

Metode

Blandt sundhedsøkonomer er koncentrationsindekset blevet en standardmetode for måling af indkomstrelateret ulighed i sundhedstatus og sundhedsydelser. Koncentrationsindekset er en generaliseret Gini-koefficient, der viser, hvordan en sundhedsvariabel (sundhedsstatus eller sundhedsydelser) er fordelt i forhold til rangordningen af en anden variabel (indkomst). Koncentrationsindekset kan grafisk udledes af koncentrationskurven, som er skitseret i figur 1. En koncentrationskurve viser den akkumulerede andel af sundhedsvariablen som en funktion af den relative indkomstrang. Hvis sundhedsvariablen er koncentreret blandt højindkomstgrupperne, vil koncentrationskurven være konveks som på figur 1a, mens kurven vil være konkav, hvis sundhedsvariablen er koncentreret blandt lavindkomstgrupperne som på figur 1b. Jo længere væk kurven er fra diagonalen, jo større ulighed. Koncentrationsindekset beregnes som det dobbelte areal mellem koncentrationskurven og diagonalen. Indekset kan variere mellem -1 og 1 og er positivt, hvis koncentrationen er blandt højindkomstgrupperne og vice versa for en koncentration blandt lavindkomstgrupperne. Indekset er 0, hvis sundhedsvariablen er ligeligt fordelt langs diagonalen, eller hvis koncentrationskurven krydser diagonalen med tilpas modsatrettede effekter.

Koncentrationsindekset har den egenskab, at individernes indkomstposition afspejles i indekset. Koncentrationsindekset inkluderer endvidere hele den samplede population – ikke kun de mest ekstreme grupper. Indekset er også følsomt overfor omfordelinger på tværs af populationen, og indeksværdien afspejler både korrelation og variation. Desuden kan koncentrationsindekset nemt estimeres med OLS-regression. Hvis den relative sundhedsvariabel, multipliceret med en konstant, regresseres på den relative indkomstrang, så vil OLS-estimatoren til den relative rang svare til koncentrationsindekset.

Koncentrationsindekset, som skitseret i figur 1, viser uligheden i sundhedsvariablen i forhold til en helt uniform fordeling. Hvis koncentrationsindekset skal vise uligheden i forhold til en anden fordeling, f.eks. hvis sundhedsydelserne skal vurderes i forhold til en behovsfordeling, må man standardisere koncentrationsindekset for de variable, som bestemmer behovet. Der er to måder at standardisere koncentrationsindekset på.

Figur 1. Eksempel på koncentrationskurver

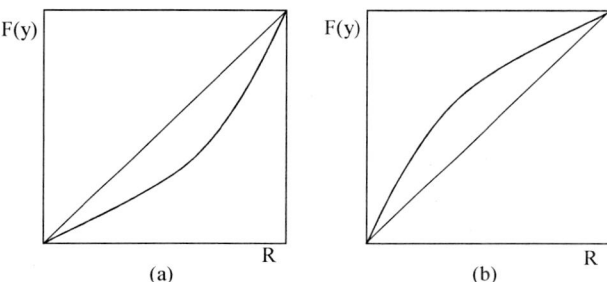

(a) Variablen y er koncentreret blandt de højere indkomstpercentiler (b) Variablen y er koncentreret blandt de lavere indkomstpercentiler.

Ved *indirekte standardisering* estimeres sundhedsvariablen på baggrund af standardiseringsvariablene, som er de variable, hvis effekt man gerne vil fjerne. Den estimerede sundhedsvariabel anvendes til at beregne et forventet koncentrationsindeks. Det standardiserede koncentrationsindeks estimeres som forskellen på det observerede og det forventede koncentrationsindeks.

Ved *direkte standardisering* udnyttes det, at sundhedsvariablen kan relateres til forskellige forklarende variable, som både kan være standardiseringsvariable og ikke-standardiseringsvariable. Relationen kan udnyttes til at dekomponere koncentrationsindekset i en komponent for hver forklarende variabel, som består af koncentrationsindekset for den forklarende variabel multipliceret med elasticiteten for sundhedsvariablen mht. den forklarende variabel. Dekompositionen viser, at en forklarende variabel påvirker den indkomstrelaterede ulighed i sundhedsvariablen, hvis der er indkomstrelateret ulighed i den pågældende variabel, og at der er en sammenhæng mellem den pågældende variabel og sundhedsvariablen. Den direkte standardisering foretages ved at fjerne komponenterne for standardiseringsvariablene fra det observerede koncentrationsindeks.

Dekompositionsmetoden kan derfor både bruges til at standardisere og til at vise hvilke determinanter, der påvirker den indkomstrelaterede ulighed i sundhedsvariablen.

Hvis sundhedsvariablen er additivt sammensat af forskellige dimensioner (sundhedsydelser består af forskellige typer af sundhedsydelser, og sundhedsstatus består af forskellige aspekter af sundhedsstatus), så kan koncentrationsindekset endvidere dekomponeres på tværs af disse dimensioner. Denne dekomposition viser hvilke dimensioner, der bidrager mest til den overordnede indkomstrelaterede ulighed i sundhedsvariablen.

Datamateriale
Datamaterialet bygger på en kombination af survey-data og registerdata. Survey-dataene består af en befolkningsundersøgelse foretaget i Fyns Amt omkring årsskiftet til 2001. 5000 personer i alderen 16-80 blev udtrukket vha. en stratificeret udtrækningsmetode fra cpr-registeret til deltagelse i en telefoninterviewundersøgelse om sundhedsstatus målt med EQ-5D og SF-36, sundhedsadfærd angående tobak, alkohol, kost og motion samt socio-demografiske og –økonomiske forhold i form af køn, alder, indkomst, uddannelse og beskæftigelsesforhold mm. Disse data blev sammenkørt med registerdata for forbrug i sundhedsydelser på somatiske hospitaler så som indlæggelser, ambulante besøg og skadestuebesøg. Fra det primære sundhedsvæsen blev der udtrukket ydelser fra almen praktiserende læge, speciallæge, fysioterapeut og tandlæge. Endvidere blev dataene sammenkørt med en database for tilskudsberettiget receptpligtigt medicin. Forbruget af sundhedsydelser, indsamlet for 2000-2001, er målt i omkostninger og approksimeret med takster, priser og honorerer.

I telefoninterviewundersøgelser er der altid personer, som af den ene eller anden grund ikke deltager. Pga. oversampling, eksternt og internt frafald kunne analyserne foretages på ca. 2900 personer.

Indkomstrelateret ulighed i forbrug af sundhedsydelser
Analyserne viste, at sundhedsydelser overordnet set er koncentreret blandt lavindkomstgrupperne. Koncentrationsindekset for de totale sundhedsomkostninger er estimeret til -0,14, hvilket er statistisk

signifikant forskelligt fra 0. Samme mønster kan man finde for de forskellige typer af sundhedsydelser, og koncentrationsindeksene er statistisk signifikante for hospitalskontakter, almen praktiserende læge og receptmedicin. En undtagelse er tandlægeydelser, som er koncentreret blandt højindkomstgrupperne.

Når koncentrationsindekset standardiseres for behov, ændres resultaterne noget. Som et *proxy* for behov er der anvendt køn, alder og sundhedsstatus. På det overordnede plan mindskes det negative koncentrationsindeks absolut og er ikke længere signifikant. For de totale sundhedsydelser ser det ikke ud til, at princippet om *lige behandling for lige behov* bliver overtrådt. Hospitalssektoren udgør en stor andel af de samlede omkostninger og er derfor den vigtigste bidragsyder til det overordnede negative koncentrationsindeks.

I den primære sektor ændres koncentrationsindeksene en del med standardiseringen for behov, således at alle koncentrationsindeksene viser en koncentration af forbruget i forhold til behovet blandt højindkomstgrupperne. Estimaterne er dog kun statistisk signifikante for de typer af sundhedsydelser, hvor der er en høj grad af brugerbetaling, nemlig for tandlægeydelser og receptmedicin. I modsætning til tidligere internationale undersøgelser, hvor Danmark også indgår, er koncentrationsindekset for ydelser ved praktiserende speciallæge lille og statistisk insignifikant.

Blandt de forklarende variable, så bidrager indkomstulighed til indkomstrelateret ulighed i forbruget af sundhedsydelser til fordel for de høje indkomstgrupper, men dette bidrag er kun statistisk signifikant for nogle typer af sundhedsydelser. Det er bl.a. insignifikant for de totale sundhedsomkostninger. For receptmedicin forklares det meste af det positive bidrag til ulighed af en uforklaret komponent, og indkomst spiller her kun en lille direkte rolle. Arbejdsmarkedet er kendt for at være tæt relateret til sundhed i Danmark, og analyserne viser også, at inaktivitet, som at være pensioneret, er en vigtig bidragsyder for ulighedsestimatet – men dog i negativ retning – dvs. til fordel for de lavere indkomstgrupper. Uddannelse, civilstand og sundhedsadfærd spiller en relativt lille direkte rolle i forklaringen af koncentrationsindeksene for indkomstrelateret ulighed i forbrug af sundhed.

Indkomstrelateret ulighed i sundhed
Resultaterne viste, at sundhed er signifikant koncentreret blandt højindkomstgrupperne. Med EQ-5D værdier som sundhedsstatusmål blev koncentrationsindekset estimeret til 0,013. Blandt de forklarende variable viste det sig, at inaktivitet på arbejdsmarkedet er en vigtig determinant i forklaringen af indkomstrelateret ulighed i sundhed. Som tidligere undersøgelser for Danmark også har vist, så forklares en meget stor del af ulighedsestimatet af pensionisters dårlige helbred samt af deres relativt dårlige indkomstforhold. Indkomstulighed spiller også en vigtig rolle for den indkomstrelaterede ulighed i sundhed. Dette er forventeligt, men i modstrid med resultater fra tidligere undersøgelser for Danmark. Demografiske variable som køn og alder bidrager negativt til ulighedsestimatet. Det betyder, at hvis man standardiserer koncentrationsindekset for socio-demografiske variable, så øges ulighedsestimatet. Uddannelse, civilstand og sundhedsadfærd spiller en relativt lille direkte rolle i forklaringen af koncentrationsindeksene for indkomstrelateret ulighed i sundhed.

Blandt de forskellige dimensioner af sundhed viste dekompositionen, at smerter og ubehag eller at have rapporteret generelle problemer med sundhed er de vigtigste faktorer i forklaringen af det overordnede ulighedsestimat.

Analyserne for ulighed i sundhed blev også udført med de generelle helbredskomponenter fra SF-36: Det fysiske helbredskomponent (PCS) og det psykiske helbredskomponent (MCS). Koncentrationsindeksene for PCS og MCS blev estimeret til henholdsvis 0,013 og 0,008. Dekomposition af EQ-5D og PCS gav næsten samme resultater, mens dekompositionen af MCS var noget anderledes, idet køn og alder bidrager positivt til uligheden, og inaktivitet på arbejdsmarkedet spiller en mindre rolle. Den komplicerede scoringsmekanisme for SF-36-helbredskomponenterne betyder dog, at fortolkningen af bidrag fra forskellige sundhedsdimensioner er svær og problematisk.

Diskussion

Afhandlingen viser, at det kan være nyttigt at anvende dekompositionsmetoden, når koncentrationsindeks bruges til at estimere indkomstrelateret ulighed i sundhedsstatus og forbrug af sundhedsydelser. Forskellige determinanter og dimensioner bidrager til det overordnede ulighedsestimat med varierende størrelser. Dekompositionsmetoden kan hjælpe med at vise forskellige faktorers modsatrettede påvirkninger og deres omfang.

I den pågældende afhandling er der dog en række forbehold, der skal tages. Først og fremmest bygger analyserne på tværsnitsdata. Derfor skal man være varsom med at fortolke forskellige relationer som kausalsammenhænge. Dekompositionsmetoden kan påpege vigtige faktorer for uligheden, men analyserne fortæller ikke, hvad mulighederne er for, at disse faktorer rent faktisk kan modificeres med policy-interventioner. Der var endvidere problemer med bortfald, idet kun 58 pct. af den udtrukne stikprøve endte med at deltage i undersøgelsen. Bortfaldsanalyser viste, at der var en tendens til underestimering af forbruget af sundhedsydelser, hvilket kunne tyde på, at datasættet muligvis ikke er helt repræsentativt for den fynske befolkning. Det er dog ikke muligt at vurdere bortfaldets betydning for ulighedsestimaternes størrelse. Ulighedsestimaternes validitet er tilmed baseret på, at sundhedsstatus opfattes ens på tværs af forskellige grupper. Selvrapporteret sundhed vil kunne variere på tværs af indkomstgrupper, hvis der er forskellige subjektive vurderinger af, hvad der er godt og dårligt helbred. Endvidere er det også et spørgsmål, om sundhedsstatus er en god *proxy* for behov. For nogle typer af sundhedsydelser vil sundhedsstatus være en bedre behovsindikator end for andre.

Indsamlingen af data er foretaget i Fyns Amt omkring årsskiftet til 2001. Der er siden gået nogle år, og en reform af det danske sundhedsvæsen er trådt i kraft. De grundlæggende principper for adgang til sundhedsydelser har dog ikke ændret sig nævneværdig, så de fleste resultater fra afhandlingen vurderes til stadigt at være kendetegnende for Fyn såvel som for resten af Danmark. De længerevarende konsekvenser af reformen samt den øgede brug af sundhedsforsikringer på arbejdsmarkedet er dog uklare, og dette peger på relevansen af fremtidig forskning om fordelingen af sundhed og sundhedsydelser i befolkningen.

Vejledning til de enkelte kapitler

Afhandlingen består af otte kapitler: Et introducerende kapitel, fire publicerede artikler, to arbejdspapirer og et afsluttende kapitel bestående af en diskussion og konklusion.

Kapitel 1 introducerer emnet. Der er et afsnit om teorier om social retfærdighed og et afsnit om den sundhedsøkonomiske tilgang til sundhedsadfærd. Derudover er der et metodemæssigt afsnit, hvor målemetoder og dekompositionsmetoder introduceres. Kapitlet afsluttes med en præsentation af datamaterialet og en kort introduktion til det danske sundhedsvæsen.

Kapitel 2 fokuserer på indkomstrelateret ulighed i receptmedicin målt med koncentrationsindeks. Medicinforbrug er repræsenteret med DDD og AUP. Horisontal ulighed er estimeret med indirekte standardisering, hvor der er anvendt en *two-part*-model til at estimere det behovsforventede forbrug på baggrund af køn, alder og sundhedstilstand. Dataene indgik uvægtede i analysen.

Kapitel 3 handler om indkomstrelateret ulighed i forbrug af sundhedsydelser. Seks typer af sundhedsydelser samt en kategori af de aggregerede sundhedsydelser indgår i analysen. Forbruget af sundhedsydelser er kvantificeret med takster, honorarer og priser (justeret så egenbetaling også indgår). Horisontal ulighed er estimeret med indirekte standardisering, hvor der er anvendt en *two-part*-model til at estimere det behovsforventede forbrug af sundhedsydelser på baggrund af køn, alder og sundhedstilstand. Ikke-standardiseringsvariable indgår i estimationen, men deres effekt er delvist neutraliseret ved at holde dem konstante. Datasættet er vægtet med de reciprokke udtrækningssandsynligheder.

I **kapitel 4** er ulighedsestimaterne standardiseret med dekompositionsmetoden. Lineære partielle effekter er approksimeret fra en *two-part*-model. Den overordnede indkomstrelaterede ulighed i forbrug af sundhedsydelser er dekomponeret i bidrag fra standardiserings- og ikke-standardiseringsvariable og i bidrag fra seks forskellige typer af sundhedsydelser. Datasættet er vægtet med de reciprokke udtrækningssandsynligheder.

Kapitel 5 fokuserer på indkomstrelateret ulighed i sundhed. Sundhedsstatus målt med EQ-5D-værdier (danske TTO-vægte) er anvendt til at operationalisere sundhed. Koncentrationsindekset for den overordnede indkomst relaterede ulighed i sundhed er dekomponeret i bidrag fra standardiserings- og ikke-standardiseringsvariable og i bidrag fra de forskellige EQ-5D-dimensioner. De partielle effekter til dekompositionen er estimeret med OLS-regression. Dataene indgik uvægtede i analysen.

I **kapitel 6** er dekomposionsteknikkerne appliceret på SF-36-helbredskomponenterne PCS og MCS. Den overordnede indkomst relaterede ulighed i sundhed, målt med PCS og MCS, er dekomponeret i bidrag fra standardiserings- og ikke-standardiseringsvariable og i bidrag fra de forskellige SF-36-dimensioner. De partielle effekter til dekompositionerne er estimeret med OLS-regression. Datasættet er vægtet med de reciprokke udtrækningssandsynligheder.

En bortfaldsanalyse præsenteres i **kapitel 7**. Her er *bias* i sundhedsforbrugsestimaterne som følge af bortfald kvantificeret ved at sammenligne respondenter og ikke-respondenter. Størrelse, retning og årsag til *bias* som følge af bortfald analyseres for to typer af datasæt: Den fynske befolkningsundersøgelse som er anvendt i afhandlingens andre analyser samt Sundheds- og sygelighedsundersøgelsen fra Statens Institut for Folkesundhed.

Afhandlingens overordnede resultater opsummeres i **kapitel 8**, hvor der også er en diskussion af undersøgelsens begrænsninger samt mulighederne for fremtidig forskning.

Ph.D.-afhandlinger og disputatser fra Det Samfundsvidenskabelige Fakultet, Syddansk Universitet:

1. Mogens Nielsen: *Finansielle nøgletals anvendelighed i statistisk baserede analytiske modeller.* Tildelt og udgivet i 1987.

2. Tage Koed Madsen: *Empirisk undersøgelse af nogle danske fremstillingsvirksomheders eksportaktiviteter.* Tildelt og udgivet i 1987.

3. Nis Jul Clausen: *Finansiering via selskabsopsplitning.* Tildelt og udgivet i 1987.

4. Niels Chr. Petersen: *The Unemployment-Health relationship - a theoretical and empirical investigation.* Tildelt og udgivet i 1987.

5. Søren Overgaard Sørensen: *Hæftelsesforholdene indenfor andelsselskabsretten.* Tildelt og udgivet i 1989.

6. Thomas Hemmer: *Regulering af eksterne regnskaber - en analyse af konsekvenser ved reduktion af valgmulighederne.* Tildelt og udgivet i 1989.

7. Jan Møller Jensen: *Familiens købsbeslutninger - Et "købscenter" perspektiv.* Tildelt og udgivet i 1990.

8. Peter Ellemann-Jensen: *Sundhedsøkonomiske aspekter af medicinsk teknologi-vurdering.* Tildelt i 1991 og udgivet i 1992.

9. Kristian Risgaard Miltersen: *A Model of the Term Structure of Interest Rates.* Tildelt i 1992 og udgivet i 1993.

10. Søren Askegaard: *Livsstilsundersøgelser: Henimod et teoretisk fundament.* Tildelt og udgivet i 1993.

11. Lars Thøger Christensen: *Marketing som organisering og kommunikation. En kulturteoretisk analyse af markedskommunikationens organisering og betydning i den marketing-orienterede virksomhed.* Tildelt og udgivet i 1993.

12. Peter Dahler-Larsen: *Fællesskabet af dem, som intet fællesskab har. En sociologisk undersøgelse af organisationskultur hinsides et integrations-perspektiv.* Tildelt og udgivet i 1993.

13. Sven Madsen: *På vej mod målet. Decentralisering og målstyring i den kommende sektor.* Udgivet på Jurist- og Økonomforbundets Forlag. Tildelt og udgivet i 1993.

14. Carsten Sørensen: *Valutakurser og nominelle rentestrukturer.* Tildelt og udgivet i 1993.

15. Ole Olesen: *Some recent studies of methods for measuring technical efficiency.* Tildelt i 1993 og udgivet i 1995.

16. Per Servais: *Internationale industrielle indkøb - i en strategisk synsvinkel.* Tildelt og udgivet i 1994.

17. Birgitte Bjørn: *Factoring - A Comparative Analysis.* Udgivet på Jurist- og Økonomforbundets Forlag. Tildelt og udgivet i 1994.

18. Jytte Larsen: *Incitamentsystemer for Kreditmedarbejdere i Pengeinstitutter.* Tildelt 1994 og udgivet i 1996.

19. Lars Thore Jensen: *Internationalisering og de danske amter.* Tildelt og udgivet i 1995.

20. Jørgen Lauridsen: *Anvendelse af regionaløkonomiske metoder i analyse af kommunal udgiftsadfærd.* Tildelt og udgivet i 1995.

21. Kristian Kidholm: *Estimation af betalingsvilje for forebyggelse af personskader i trafikulykker.* Tildelt og udgivet i 1995.

22. Erling Dalgaard Andersen: *Solution of Linear and Convex Optimization Problems with Emphasis on Interior Point Methods.* Tildelt og udgivet i 1996.

23. Niels Ejersbo: *Den kommunale forvaltning under omstilling - En organisationsteoretisk analyse af effekter af forvaltningsændringer ud fra et ledelsesperspektiv og et læringsperspektiv.* Tildelt og udgivet i 1996.

24. Hans Frimor: *Renegotiation and Asymmetric Information in Multi Period Agencies.* Tildelt og udgivet i 1996.

25. Lars K. Langkilde: *Uncertainty, Information and Health Technology.* Tildelt og udgivet i 1997.

26. Jie Zhang: *The Economic Relations Between the European Union and East Asia.* Tildelt og udgivet i 1997.

27. Per Østergaard: *Træk af marketing disciplinens epistemologiske udvikling: En periodisering af amerikansk marketingteoris historie med fokus på accepten af de kvalitative metoder.* Tildelt i 1996 og udgivet i 1997.

28. Morten Balle Hansen: *En organisationssociologisk undersøgelse af struktureringen af kommunaldirektørens arbejde med udgangspunkt i et aktør-strukturperspektiv.* Tildelt og udgivet i 1997.

29. Claus Munk: *Optimal Consumption/Portfolio Policies and Contingent Claims Pricing and Hedging in Incomplete Markets.* Tildelt og udgivet i 1997.

30. Jørgen Clausen: *Sundhedsøkonomiske aspekter vedrørende offentlige medicintilskud og finansieringen af lægemidler.* Tildelt i 1997 og udgivet i 1998.

31. Dorte Gyrd-Hansen: *Modelling the cost-effectiveness of cancer screening in Denmark.* Tildelt i 1997 og udgivet i 1998.

32. Jan Guldager Jørgensen: *Regional integration og multinationale virksomheder.* Tildelt og udgivet i 1998.

33. Eva Ulrichsen Draborg: *Effektevaluering af sundhedsinformation - med impirisk analyse af et præoperativt patientinformationsprogram og af en oplysningskampagne mod narkotikamisbrug.* Tildelt og udgivet i 1998.

34. Annie Gaardsted Frandsen: *Landspolitik eller lokalpolitik? Et studie af danske kommunalvalg.* Tildelt og udgivet i 1998.

35. Bo Eriksen: *Core Competence: Linking Strategy and Organization.* Tildelt i 1997 og udgivet i 1998.

36. Tim Jeppesen: *Institutional Arrangements for Environmental policy in a Federal System - with Applications to the European Union.* Tildelt og udgivet i 1998.

37. Anders Damgaard: *Optimal Portfolio Choice and Utility Based Option Pricing in Markets with Transaction Costs.* Tildelt og udgivet i 1999.

38. Roger Buch Jensen: *Lokale partiorganisationer.* Tildelt i 1998 og udgivet i 2000.

39. Jan Paludan Warhuus: *Risk and Uncertainty in Entrepreneurial Decision-Making and Resource Acquisition.* Tildelt og udgivet i 1999.

40. Anne Flemmert Jensen: *Acknowledging and Consuming Fashion in the Era After 'Good Taste' - From 'the Beautiful to 'the Hideous'.* Tildelt i 1998 og udgivet i 1999.

41. Fabian Faurholt Csaba: *Designs of the Retail Entertainment Complex. Marketing, Space and the Mall of America.* Tildelt og udgivet i 1999.

42. Jan Stentoft Arlbjørn: *A Comparative Logistical Analysis: A Search for a Contingence Theory. - The Manufacturer's Perspective*. Tildelt i 1999 og udgivet i 2000.

43. Rikke Berg: *Den gode politiker. Et studie af politiske ledelsesværdier i kommunerne*. Tildelt i 1999 og udgivet i 2000.

44. Teit Lüthje: *Udenrigshandel med halvfabrikata. Udvikling af ½ teorier til forklaring af udenrigshandel med halvfabrikata samt applicering heraf på den danske udenrigshandel med halvfabrikata*. Tildelt i 1999 og udgivet i 2000.

45. Carsten Lynge Jensen: *Behavioural Modelling of Fishermen in the EU*. Tildelt i 1999 og udgivet i 2000.

46. Ulrik Kjær: *Kommunalbestyrelsens sammensætning - rekruttering og repræsentation i dansk kommunalpolitik*. Tildelt og udgivet i 2000.

47. Vibeke Normann Andersen: *Reformer i folkeskolen. Relationer mellem aktører i det lokale skolefelt*. Tildelt og udgivet i 2000.

48. Thorbjørn Knudsen: *The Firm's environmental and competitive strategy*. Tildelt i 2000 og udgivet i 2001.

49. Ulla Slothuus: *Economic Evaluation in Health Care: Issues in Costing and Willingness to Pay Measurements With Applications to Arthritis and Heart Disease*. Tildelt i 2000 og udgivet i 2001.

50. Christian Kronborg Andersen: *Health Economics of dementia. Issues on the estimation of cost functions and modelling costs and health outcomes of dementia interventions*. Tildelt og udgivet i 2001.

51. Camilla Jensen: *Foreign direct investment and technological change in Polish manufacturing, 1989-98*. Tildelt i 2000 og udgivet i 2001.

52. Jens Bøgetoft Christensen: *Livsverden og kultur. Ansatser til en fænomenologisk baseret organisationsforståelse.* Tildelt i 2001 og udgivet 2002.

53. Lars Thording: *Professionalism and Marketing. An orientational Approach.* Tildelt i 2001 og udgivet i 2002.

54. Frank Jensen: *Essays in Management of Fisheries under Imperfect Information.* Tildelt i 2001 og udgivet i 2002.

55. Erik S. Rasmussen: *Internationaliseringsprocesser i hurtigt internationaliserede danske små og mellemstore produktionsvirksomheder.* Tildelt i 2001 og udgivet i 2002.

56. Christian Riis Flor: *Dynamic Capital Structure.* Tildelt i 2002 og udgivet i 2003.

57. Mette Hansen: *Applying Financial Economics to Life and Pension Insurance.* Tildelt i 2002 og udgivet i 2003.

58. Klaus Levinsen: *Unges politiske værdier - i et generationsperspektiv.* Tildelt i 2002 og udgivet i 2003.

59. Derek Beach: *Bringing negotiations back into the study of European integration.* Tildelt i 2002 og udgivet i 2003.

60. Shahamak Rezaei: *Erhvervsdynamik blandt indvandrere: Selverhverv og netværksrelationer - blokering eller afsæt for socioøkonomisk mobilitet?* Tildelt i 2002 og udgivet i 2004.

61. Dorthe Døjbak: *An examination of the Relationship between Excecutive Cognition Orientation, Strategic Decision-Making, and Firm Performance.* Tildelt og udgivet i 2003.

62. Mette Sicard Filtenborg: *Building Strategic Partnerships in Euro-polity Affairs.* Tildelt og udgivet i 2003.

63. Jesper Piihl: *Ledelseskoncepters rolle i organiseringsprocesser.* Tildelt og udgivet i 2003.

64. Niels Grünbaum: *Industriel kundetilfredshed?* Tildelt og udgivet i 2003.

65. Jeanette Lemmergaard: *Tolerance for Ambiguity. The Intersection between Ethnical Climate, Psychological Climate, and Ethnic Diversity.* Tildelt i 2003 og udgivet i 2004.

66. Mickael Bech: *Choice of Hospital Reimbursement Scheme: Incentives and Tradeoffs.* Tildelt i 2003 og udgivet 2004.

67. Dannie Kjeldgaard: *Consumption and the Global Youth Segment. Peripheral Positions, Central Immersion.* Tildelt i 2003 og udgivet i 2004.

68. Illiana Kohler: *Adult and Old-Age Mortality Dynamics in Bulgaria and Russia.* Tildelt i 2002 og udgivet i 2007.

69. Ann Højbjerg Clarke: *Segmentation of industrial markets and determining product lines for product development.* Tildelt i 2002 og udgivet i 2004.

70. Kasper Møller Hansen: *Deliberative Democracy and Opinion Formation.* Tildelt og udgivet i 2004.

71. Thomas Gulløv: *Organizational Adaptation.* Tildelt og udgivet i 2004.

72. Marianne Figge Stein: *A Cross-Cultural Comparison of Advertising and Attitudes to Advertising in Denmark and the United States.* Tildelt og udgivet i 2004.

73. Anna Lund Jepsen: *Consumer Search for Information on the Internet.* Tildelt og udgivet i 2004.

74. Peter Bindslev Iversen: *Why Not Take Wise Decisions?* Tildelt og udgivet i 2004.

75. Kennet Lynggaard: *The Common Agriculture Policy and The Dynamics of Institutional Change.* Tildelt i 2004 og udgivet i 2005.

76. Gitte Meyer: *Offentlig fornuft? Videnskab, journalistik og samfundsmæssig praksis.* Tildelt i 2004 og udgivet i 2005.

77. Lars Jensen: *LDR modeller.* Tildelt i 2004 og udgivet i 2005.

78. Lone Grønbæk Kronbak: *Essays on Strategic Interaction and Behaviour among Agents in Fisheries.* Tildelt i 2004 og udgivet i 2005.

79. Max Nielsen: *Linkages between Seafood Markets, Fisheries Management and Trade Liberalisation: Theory and Applications.* Tildelt i 2004 og udgivet i 2005.

80. Erik Lindebo: *Managing Capacity in Fisheries.* Tildelt i 2004 og udgivet i 2005.

81. Ole Friis: *Formuebaseret regnskab. Er det bedre?* Tildelt og udgivet i 2005.

82. Bodil Stilling Blichfeldt: *On Brand and Line Extensions.* Tildelt i 2004 og udgivet i 2006.

83. Kent Wickstrøm Jensen: *Knowledge-Integration Networks in Product Development.* Tildelt i 2005 og udgivet i 2006.

84. Kim U. Wittrup Jensen: *Measurement and Valuation of Health-Related Quality of Life.* Tildelt i 2005 og udgivet i 2006.

85. Sanne Wøhlk: *Contributions to Arc Routing.* Tildelt i 2005 og udgivet i 2006.

86. Hans Eibe Sørensen: *On Market Orientation. Development and empirical validation of two symmetric component measures of market orientation.* Tildelt i 2005 og udgivet i 2006.

87. Majbritt Rostgaard Evald: *Brugen og betydningen af personlige netværk i udviklingen af højteknologiske virksomheder inden for en koncerninkubator.* Tildelt i 2005 og udgivet i 2006.

88. Edlira Gjonça: *Socio-Economic Determinants of Longevity in Denmark, England and Wales – A Comparative Study.* Tildelt i 2003 og udgivet i 2007.

89. Poul Skov Dahl: *Standardisering som reguleringsform. En analyse af KL som meta-organisation og standardsætter på ældreområdet.* Tildelt og udgivet i 2006.

90. Tipparat Pongthanapanich: *Coastal Land Use Management in Thailand: Policy Development Tools for a Better Environment.* Tildelt og udgivet i 2007.

91. Jean-Paul de Cros Péronard: *Communication, Convergence, and Contradictions. The Emergent Culture of Inter-Organizational Networks.* Tildelt i 2006 og udgivet i 2007.

92. Maciej Wilga: *Approaching a "Pluribus Unum" in EU High Politics. Explaining the CFSP Emergence and Institutional Development from Maastricht to the 2003/4 IGC.* Tildelt og udgivet i 2007.

93. Troels Martin Range: *Exact Solution of Resource Constrained Routing Problems using Branch-Price-and-Cut.* Tildelt i 2006 og udgivet i 2007.

94. Finn Olesen: *Rundt om "The General Theory"- en teorihistorisk belysning* Tildelt og udgivet i 2007.

95. Jens Kjærsgaard: *Fisheries mangement: incorporating multiple objectives*. Tildelt i 2007 og udgivet i 2008.

96. Jens Ringsmose: *Frihedens assurancepræmie. Danmark, NATO og forsvarsbudgetterne*. Tildelt i 2007 og udgivet i 2008.

97. Simon Lysbjerg Hansen: *Three topics in asset allocation and asset pricing*. Tildelt i 2007 og udgivet i 2008.

98. Jens Gundgaard: *The Distribution of Health and Health Care*. Tildelt i 2007 og udgivet i 2008.

Følgende disputatser har været forsvaret ved Det Samfundsvidenskabelige Fakultet ved Odense Universitet efter 1. januar 1987:

1. Peter Ove Christensen: *Asymmetric Information, Efficient Resource Allocation and Moral Hazard in Capital Markets*. Tildelt og udgivet i 1990.

2. Carsten A. Koch: *Decision, Transaction, Law and Contract. A Study in Transaction Cost Economics on an Individualistic Basis, with Emphasis on the Economic Rationale of Contracts*. Tildelt i 1997.

3. Tage Koed Madsen: *Virksomheders eksport og internationale konkurrenceevne*. Tildelt i 1997.